Patient Management Skills for Dental Assistants and Hygienists

BARBARA D. INGERSOLL, Ph.D.

West Virginia University
School of Dentistry

48630

APPLETON-CENTURY-CROFTS/Norwalk, Connecticut

To Tom, with gratitude

86 87 88 89 90/10 9 8 7 6 5 4 3 2 1

Editorial/production supervision and interior design: Paul Spencer
Cover design: Lundgren Graphics, Ltd.
Manufacturing buyer: John Hall

Prentice-Hall International (UK) Limited, *London*
Prentice-Hall of Australia Pty. Limited, *Sydney*
Prentice-Hall Canada Inc., *Toronto*
Prentice-Hall Hispanoamericana, S.A., *Mexico*
Prentice-Hall of India Private Limited, *New Delhi*
Prentice-Hall of Japan, Inc., *Tokyo*
Prentice-Hall of Southeast Asia Pte. Ltd., *Singapore*
Editora Prentice-Hall do Brasil, Ltda., *Rio de Janeiro*
Whitehall Books Limited, *Wellington, New Zealand*

ISBN 0-8385-7779-2

Library of Congress Cataloging in Publication Data

Ingersoll, Barbara D., (date)
    Patient management skills for dental assistants
and hygienists.

    Includes bibliographies and index.
    1. Dentistry—Psychological aspects. 2. Dentist
and patient. 3. Dentistry—Practice. 4. Dental
assistants. 5. Dental hygienists. I. Title. [DNLM:
1. Dental Assistants. 2. Dental Care—psychology.
3. Dental Hygienists. 4. Professional-Patient
Relations. WU 90 I47p]
RK53.I54 1986   617.6'0233   85-6551
ISBN 0-8385-7779-2

Printed in the United States of America

Contents

Section IV   ADHERENCE TO HEALTH CARE REGIMENS

Section V   SPECIAL PATIENTS, SPECIAL PROBLEMS

Preface

In the past several years, much has been said about the stress associated with the practice of the oral health professions and about the high rate of "burn-out" among dental professionals. Many factors bear on the situation, but one that appears to be of particular significance is the frequency with which the dental professional encounters difficulty in the area of patient management.

Patients who do not follow instructions, who cancel or fail to come in for appointments, or who exhibit disproportionate fear of dental treatment have long been cited by dentists as *the* major source of job-related stress. As dental assistants and dental hygienists assume increasing responsibilities for patient care, it is likely that they, too, will experience increasing patient-management problems and difficulties.

Such issues have received growing attention, not only from those within the oral health professions but also from behavioral scientists who have directed research efforts toward resolving many of these problems. Scientific investigations in such areas as dental fear, coping with the stress of dental treatment, and adherence to preventive regimens have advanced our understanding of these issues and contain important implications for the practice of dental hygiene and dental assisting.

This book draws upon the results of this research for assistance with a variety of patient-management problems. Although many questions remain to be answered, the results of scientific investigations can help dental assistants and dental hygienists to develop practical and effective approaches to dealing with many of the patient-management problems they encounter.

CONTRIBUTORS

Christina B. DeBiase, B.S.D.H., M.A.
West Virginia University School of Dentistry

Sanford J. Fenton, D.D.S., M.D.S.
West Virginia University School of Dentistry

Michael J. Geboy, Ph.D.
Georgetown University School of Dentistry

1

Expanded Roles, Expanded Responsibilities

Almost a quarter of a century ago, it was noted that "dentistry today, and certainly in the future, finds itself in a position that relies heavily upon the services of its auxiliaries."[1] The increased utilization of dental assistants and dental hygienists has been one of the most significant trends in modern dentistry. As the number of assistants and hygienists has grown, there has been a thrust toward expanding the professional functions of these groups. Although this movement has encountered many obstacles and has not yet achieved complete success, it is undeniable that the duties and responsibilities of dental assistants and hygienists have broadened considerably.

With the expansion of professional roles comes a corresponding need for increased skills and expertise. At least where technical expertise is concerned, a recent survey conducted by the American Dental Association suggests that the public is well-satisfied with the performance of assistants and hygienists.[2] When a large group of dental patients was asked whether they were satisfied with the duties performed by the auxiliary during their last dental visit, an overwhelming 98 percent described themselves as satisfied.

But dentistry consists of much more than the delivery of technical services. Surrounding every oral cavity there is a human being with a complex and unique assortment of hopes, fears, expectations, beliefs, emotions, and behavior. Dental professionals often find that the task of understanding and interacting with this human being—"the person behind the teeth"—is their most demanding professional challenge.

Interpersonal factors are an enormously important component of the health care process, and the relationship between provider and patient has been described as the professional's most valuable tool. Patients often base their judgement of you, the professional, on such things as your apparent warmth, interest, and concern for them. Because the provider-patient relationship and the communication skills necessary to establish and maintain this relationship underlie all successful approaches to patient management, these topics are addressed in the next three chapters, before specific management strategies for particular problems are discussed.

It is unfortunate that there has been very little research directly related to the interpersonal aspects of dental hygiene and dental assisting. We know, however, that dentists often perceive this area as problematic. Surveys show that dentists are most dissatisfied with those aspects of their practice that have to do with helping people.[3] When dentists are asked to identify sources of stress in practice, they most frequently describe patient-management problems.[4] The specific patient-management problems listed in Table 1-1 are among those most frequently cited as troublesome.[5]

As the table shows—and as we might have anticipated—the most frequently reported problem is dental fear. Fear, which plays a major role in avoidance of dental treatment, is also a significant factor in broken or cancelled appointments. It is clear that the competent dental professional must be knowledgeable about dental fear and skilled in working with fearful patients. Dental fear and avoidance are discussed in detail in Chapter 5. Promising new approaches to reducing dental fear and stress are described in Chapter 6.

Dental professionals, who know that dental caries and periodontal disease can be prevented if patients comply with preventive recommendations and instructions for home care, are likely to be quite frustrated by patients who do not follow advice. Of concern, too, are patients who fail to keep recall appointments and who seek care only in emer-

TABLE 1-1 Patient-management Problems Reported
by a National Sample of Practicing Dentists.

Problem	% Reporting Problem
Fear	87
Broken, cancelled, late appointments	76
Not motivated for oral hygiene	76
Do not follow treatment instructions	75
Disruptive or uncooperative children	59
Explaining treatment	46
Parents of child patients	39

From Ingersoll, Ingersoll, McCutcheon, and Seime, 1979.

gency situations. These issues are particularly relevant to hygienists and assistants, who have assumed increasing responsibility for instructing patients in proper home care procedures and for persuading them to comply with preventive recommendations. Various strategies to educate and motivate patients are discussed and critically evaluated in Chapters 7 and 8.

Children who are uncooperative during dental treatment pose special problems, because fearful, disruptive behavior interferes with efficient delivery of safe, high-quality care. Factors that contribute to the child's reaction to the dental experience are discussed in Chapter 9. Methods that have been successfully used to reduce fear and uncooperative behavior and to promote positive attitudes toward dentistry are also described.

At the other end of the spectrum from the child patient is the geriatric patient. The elderly represent the fastest-growing segment of our population; as their numbers increase, there is a corresponding increase in the demand for oral health care. Treatment of the elderly patient is complicated by many factors, including chronic diseases and the infirmities of old age. Some of the special needs of this group are discussed in Chapter 10.

Handicapped patients constitute another group that the dental professional can expect to encounter more frequently. In the past, the person with a physical or mental disability was more likely to be isolated at home or even in an institution. Now, as these individuals are integrated into the mainstream of our society, they are appearing in greater numbers in the dental office. Practical suggestions for working with the disabled are provided in Chapter 11.

THE ROLE OF RESEARCH IN PATIENT MANAGEMENT

The professional literature on dentistry, dental hygiene, and dental assisting is filled with suggestions for dealing with patient-management problems. On the subject of the fearful patient alone, for example, the number of articles describing methods for management is staggering. Few of these methods, however, are backed by any sort of proof that they are effective. They are based, for the most part, on "armchair theorizing" or on anecdotes from the author's professional experience. Such suggestions can, of course, be useful, but they can also confuse more than they clarify. When, as often happens, conflicting recommendations appear, how is the reader to decide which method is more effective, or, indeed, whether either method is effective at all?

Too often, ineffective management strategies have been recommended, adopted by practitioners, and passed on to others—especially students—as established fact. There has even been widespread adoption of methods that are not only ineffective but actually counterproductive; an example is the use of "voice control" and physical restraint with child patients—tactics which have recently been shown to result in *increases* in fearful, disruptive behavior (see Chapter 9).

Only when methods of patient management are based on the results of careful scientific investigation can we feel confident in adopting them for use with our patients. In recent years, increased interest and attention have been focused on the scientific study of such issues as provider-patient interaction and the resolution of patient-management problems. In systematic programs of research, a variety of methods have been evaluated under strictly controlled conditions. The results have shed new light on old problems and have provided us with the means to select the most efficient, effective methods to deal with these problems.

This book is based, as much as possible, on knowledge gained through research. It is particularly unfortunate that most of this research has been directed toward the dentist, because the patient management responsibilities of the hygienist and assistant are often as great as—in some cases, greater than—those of the dentist. There is considerable overlap, however, in the patient-management problems encountered by all three professional groups, so it is appropriate to draw on this body of research as the basis for this book.

REFERENCES

1. Green, E.J., and Comisarow, R.W. Work motivation and job perception as applied to a group of dental hygienists. *Dental Hygiene* 2:114, 1971.

2. American Dental Association, Bureau of Economic and Behavioral Research. Dental habits and opinions of the public: Results of a 1978 survey. Chicago: American Dental Association, 1979.

3. Burge, J.R., Ayer, W.A., and Borkman, T. Job satisfaction among dentists. IADR Abstract #1016. *Journal of Dental Research*, Special Issue A, Vol. 57, p. 329, 1978.

4. Godwin, W.C., Stark, D.D., Green, T.G., and Koran, A. Identification of sources of stress in practice by recent dental graduates. *Journal of Dental Education* 45:220, 1981.

5. Ingersoll, B.D., Ingersoll, T.G., McCutcheon, W.R., and Seime, R.J. Behavioral dimensions of dental practice: A national survey. Unpublished manuscript, West Virginia University School of Dentistry, Morgantown, West Virginia, 1979.

2

The Provider-Patient Alliance

When most people think of the health care process, their thoughts turn to scientific knowledge, technical procedures, and pharmacological agents. Few include the provider-patient relationship as an integral component of the health care process. Yet interpersonal interaction is as much a part of all health care as the technical procedures performed or the medications prescribed. In fact, evidence suggests that interpersonal factors can actually be even *more* important than other aspects of the health care process. For example, researchers have found direct links between the quality of the caregiver-patient relationship and the so-called placebo effect—the effect that results from a substance or procedure that is known to have no specific therapeutic relationship to the condition for which it is administered.

The placebo effect is an important component of all medical and dental treatment and of all medications. Even a drug as pharmacologically active as morphine has a placebo component: Researchers estimate that about half of the effects of this potent drug may be placebo effects.[1] Although many people mistakenly believe that placebo effects are "all in the patient's head," placebos can actually produce measurable physiological effects, including changes in corticosteroid levels.[2]

How does the placebo effect work? The process is not yet fully understood, but many researchers agree that it is related to the patient's belief that something is being done for him and to his expectation of relief.* These beliefs depend, to a great extent, on the patient's trust in the caregiver who prescribes the drug or treatment, the warmth displayed by the professional, and the enthusiasm with which the professional suggests that relief is to be expected.

It is clear, then, that the quality of the provider-patient relationship can actually have significant effects on the outcome of treatment. There are other benefits, as well, for both patient and provider. When the relationship between patient and provider is characterized by mutual respect and trust, all of the following result:

The patient's anxiety and apprehension are significantly reduced. Fear of dental treatment is very common—so much so that when dentists are asked to describe their most troublesome patient-management problems, fear is cited most frequently.[3] The fearful patient requires additional chair time for even the most routine procedures;[4] he is also much more likely than the nonfearful patient to break or cancel an appointment.[5] Thus, the fearful patient is a problem from an economic perspective as well as from a humane point of view.

Structured methods for reducing dental fear will be discussed in Chapter 6. It is important to emphasize here, however, that few of these formal approaches are likely to be effective in the absence of a good caregiver-patient relationship.

The patient is more likely to pay his bills on time. The problem of fee collection is also widespread in dentistry: In a recent national survey, almost three-quarters of the respondents cited this as a source of concern.[3] It is a mistake to consider fee collection as a problem of concern only to the dentist—after all, if the practice does not prosper, neither will the members of the dental team. In fact, it is a mistake even to view fee collection as simply a business management issue, since there are indications that often the provider-patient relationship lies at the heart of the problem. When patients believe they have been treated unfairly or impersonally, they often resort to nonpayment of their dental bills as a means of retaliating against the dental team. Conversely, when the provider-patient relationship is sound, the patient is more likely to pay his bills and to do so promptly. The wise business manager knows that good business management depends on good people management.

The patient speaks highly of the practitioner and the staff and recommends them to his friends. In a survey conducted by the American Dental Association, 42 percent of the respondents reported that they selected a dental practice based on recommendations from friends,

---

*The masculine pronoun has been used throughout this book to refer to the patient, in order to avoid awkward phrasing and to improve readability.

neighbors, and associates.[6] Referrals, of course, are important to any dental practice, from the new and struggling to the well-established.

The patient is more likely to remember and follow instructions and recommendations. Dental professionals are all too familiar with patients who pay no heed to instructions and recommendations concerning their oral health care. Such patients were cited as a problem by three-quarters of the respondents in a national survey of practicing dentists, many of whom described the problem as especially vexing. As one frustrated respondent wrote, "It's like talking to a wall!"[3]

In Chapter 8 we will discuss ways in which patients can be helped to assume greater responsibility for their own oral health. The provider-patient relationship, however, is the essential foundation for all preventive efforts.

The patient is less likely to sue. Dental malpractice claims are increasing rapidly—perhaps even faster than medical malpractice claims. In just one four-year period, for example, the number of malpractice claims submitted to a dental insurance company serving California dentists rose from 367 claims a year to 520 claims a year.[7] As a result, the cost of dental malpractice insurance in California rose 64 percent in the lower-risk categories and as much as 113 percent in the higher-risk categories. The cost of malpractice insurance has also risen for dental hygienists, and hygienists are increasingly likely to be named as code-fendants and even primary defendants.[8]

Why are patients suing health care professionals more frequently now than they have in the past? Experts suggest several reasons, including patients' unrealistic expectations as to what modern dentistry can accomplish, and contingent fee arrangements under which the patient does not pay the attorney's fee unless a financial settlement is reached.[9] One of the most significant factors, however, appears to be the quality of the relationship between patient and provider. One authority, for example, believes that patients resent what they perceive as impersonal care in large, multi-chair offices where they might be treated by several different persons in the course of a single visit.[10]

"Prevention," states one writer, "is the best defense in avoiding a malpractice suit." The writer stresses the importance of keeping accurate records and also notes:

> The value of good public relations should not be underestimated. Spending a few minutes socializing with patients; giving samples of home care products; taking time to give thorough instructions and allowing the patient to practice; letting the patient know you care about the patient's progress; scheduling adequate time for all procedures without long waits for the patient; calling patients the day after surgery or long scaling procedures; and communicating

real concern to all patients will go a long way toward preventing the hostility that underlies so many suits.[9]

Good ideas and good advice—for all oral health professionals!

Finally, in addition to all of these advantages gained from a good provider-patient relationship, the provider receives direct benefits—intangible but very real—in terms of increased job satisfaction. The oral health professions are demanding and often stressful, but the rewards of working effectively with people can be great. In fact, when a group of dental hygienists were asked what they liked most about the practice of their profession, "working with people" was the most common response. Results of this survey suggest that dental hygienists, as a group, tend to be warm, friendly, caring people who enjoy being with others.[11]

It is difficult to generalize from this small survey, but there is reason to believe that many dentists would agree with the findings. It is not uncommon for dentists to look to the other members of the team to provide an atmosphere of warmth, caring, and support in the office and the operatory. Many dentists simply explain, "They are better at it than I am." One well-known dentist was quoted as follows:

> People who are most qualified and skilled in communicating and in dealing with patients are those who are least technically oriented or administratively preoccupied. That's going to be the person in the auxiliary role. They are more likely to hear what patients say and understand what patients feel than is the dentist. Perhaps the more insulated the dentist is—the less he says—the better off the team is in some regard. The dentist must have the philosophy, but the dental auxiliaries have an opportunity he doesn't have.[12]

In summary, attention to the quality of the provider-patient relationship yields benefits to you, the provider, as well as to your patients. Dental hygienists and dental assistants are in an advantageous position for developing good rapport and sound relationships with their patients. The following sections will focus on the specific skills that contribute to relationship enhancement.

REFERENCES

1. Beecher, H.K. *Measurement of subjective responses: Quantitative effects of drugs.* New York: Oxford University Press, 1959.
2. Gryll, S.L., and Katahn, M. Situational factors contributing to the placebo effect. *Psychopharmacology* 57:253, 1978.
3. Ingersoll, B.D., Ingersoll, T.G., McCutcheon, W.R., and Seime, R.J. Behavioral dimensions of dental practice: A national survey. Unpublished manuscript, West Virginia University School of Dentistry, 1979.

4. Filewich, R.J., Jackson, E., and Shore, H. Effects of dental fear on efficiency of routine dental procedures. Paper presented at the meeting of the International Association for Dental Research, Chicago, March, 1981.

5. Kleinknecht, R.A. Dental fear assessment. In *Behavioral dentistry: Proceedings of the First National Conference*, edited by B. Ingersoll, R. Seime, and W. McCutcheon. Morgantown, W.Va.: West Virginia University, 1977.

6. American Dental Association, Bureau of Economic and Behavioral Research. Dental habits and opinions of the public: Results of a 1978 survey. Chicago, Ill.: American Dental Association, 1979.

7. Fat, K. The dental malpractice premium problem. *Journal of the California Dental Association* 3:8, 1975.

8. Zinman, E. Paper presented at the meeting of the Northern California State Dental Hygienists' Association, October, 1975. Cited in Paige, B.E. Malpractice: An overview for the dental hygienist. *Dental Hygiene* 51:167, 1977.

9. Paige, B.E. Malpractice: An overview for the dental hygienist. *Dental Hygiene* 51:167, 1977.

10. Morris, W.O. You're making too much of malpractice. *Dental Management* 15:12, 1975.

11. Dental hygiene manpower survey. Unpublished report, Dental Health Center, Public Health Service of the Department of Health, Education, and Welfare. San Francisco, Calif., 1972. Cited in McAdams, W.J.C. Reasons dental hygienists dislike their practice. *Dental Hygiene* 50:563, 1976.

12. Reed, O.K. 80's Practice management: The form and function of tomorrow's practice. Panel discussion, *Journal of the American Dental Association* 103:16, 1981.

3

Verbal Communication: Speaking and Listening Skills

The provider's ability to communicate effectively with patients is the basis of a successful provider-patient relationship. Communication can be defined as the process through which information is obtained from and imparted to other people. This definition is deceptively simple, however; the process of communication is really quite complex. Whenever we are in contact with another person, communication occurs. We cannot *not* communicate; even if we do not speak, we communicate through our silence. Nor should we think of communication only in terms of verbal behavior, for we also communicate a great deal to others through gestures, expressions, and movement. In fact, many anthropologists believe that gestures constituted the earliest means of human communication. Even our clothing and hairstyle and the way in which we arrange our physical space convey information to others.

Those who study communication usually divide the communication process into *encoding processes* and *decoding processes. Encoding* refers to the process of putting thoughts, ideas, and emotions into a form that can be observed by others. These internal events are the *message* of the communication. *Decoding* refers to the process by which we receive these messages and attach meaning to them. Although both encoding and decoding involve nonverbal behavior as well as verbal behavior, we will emphasize verbal communication in the following sections. Nonverbal communication will be discussed in the next chapter.

THE ENCODING PROCESS: SPEAKING SKILLS

I know you believe you understand what you think I said, but I'm not sure that you realize that what you heard is not what I meant.

Skill in sending clear messages is an essential part of good communication; as this popular quote illustrates, problems often arise when messages are ambiguous. Imprecise or careless use of language is a major factor contributing to unclear messages. Although language is, by definition, a shared symbol system, there are individual differences in the ways in which words are interpreted. Meaning resides not in the words themselves, but in the people who use the words. Because people have different sets of life experiences, the associations that certain words have for them can vary widely.

Poor speaking habits and nervous mannerisms can also interfere with the listener's ability to decode the speaker's messages. Consider the following examples:

The Decorator: Well, you know, Mrs. Benson, it's like—I mean, you know, if you would just—like, well, take better care, you know. . . .

The Decorator festoons every sentence with unnecessary verbal clutter. This distracting habit makes it difficult for the listener to concentrate on ideas and to extract meaning from what the speaker says.

The Speedster: HelloMr.SmithIt'snicetoseeyouHowareyoutoday?Justcomein andhaveaseatandwecangetstarted.

The Speedster always sounds rushed. Speaking too quickly and slurring words increases the risk of misunderstanding. Rapid-fire speech also produces feelings of tension, anxiety, and urgency in the listener. Needless to say, these are the very emotions we wish to minimize in the dental operatory.

The Screamer: HI, MR. HARNER! GOOD TO SEE YOU! HOW ARE YOU TODAY?

When the Screamer is on the scene, rafters ring and glasses shatter. So do people's nerves. A loud voice is often associated with fear, anger, and excitement. Conversely, a soft tone is soothing and relaxing, and is more effective for conveying warmth and concern.

The Mumbler: Mr. Jackson, how often do you (mumble) when you (murmur)? You know, it's really better if you (mmmph).

It is annoying to patients and colleagues to have to strain to hear what is said. Speaking too softly and looking away from the listener while speaking are behaviors that often accompany mumbling.

The Teeny Bopper: Oh, wow, Mr. Evans. What a bummer! I'll just bet you were sure ticked off!

While it is not necessary to sound stuffy or stilted, excessive use of slang detracts from a professional image. Professionals sometimes go to the opposite extreme and, in an attempt to sound professional and knowledgeable, pepper their speech with jargon. Technical terms facilitate communication among the members of a profession, but the use of a great deal of jargon with patients or others who are not familiar with the terms results in feelings of confusion and even hostility.

If you suspect that your speaking habits resemble any of those described above, it is certainly worthwhile to listen to yourself on tape. People are often unpleasantly surprised the first time they hear their own voices played back to them. A common reaction is, "I don't sound like that!" However, even inexpensive portable tape recorders reproduce speech sounds fairly accurately, so the way one sounds on tape is very similar to the way one sounds to the world.

The dental professional's use of language is also a major factor in professional-patient communication. Your choice of words can enhance or detract from your professional image. Words and phrases like *fix* and *dental work* sound less professional than *repair* or *restore* and *dental treatment*.[1] Similarly, *restoration* is preferable to *filling, primary tooth* sounds better than *baby tooth*, and Mrs. Jones would rather hear herself called a *regular patient* than an *old patient*.[1]

Most dental professionals agree that it is important to avoid words with frightening or threatening connotations when talking with patients. Thus, it is suggested that the following words be avoided:[2]

Cut
Drill
Scrape
Chisel
Knife

The phrase *remove a tooth* is recommended instead of *pull a tooth*, and *prepare a tooth* instead of *grind down a tooth*.

While we acknowledge that the dental professional must meet very high standards of precision and exactness in technical work, we seldom recognize the need for precision in our use of language, especially in interactions with patients. Unfortunately, it is probably a good bet that if a word or phrase can be interpreted in more than one way, it will be. For example, what does the term *fairly expensive* mean to you? Very little, of course, unless you have additional information about the item or service in question and the standard of comparison employed.

Other words that can easily be misunderstood include *much, a little, some, soon,* and *quickly.* Remember that what seems like *just a little while* to you might seem like eternity to the patient in the chair. To avoid unnecessary confusion and misunderstanding, strive for precision in your speech.

Minimizing Listener Defensiveness

You have probably observed that while some patients respond to you in a trusting, comfortable fashion shortly after they meet you, others seem suspicious and defensive from the moment they enter the operatory. Past learning experiences influence whether a person will generally be inclined to trust others quickly and easily, or will tend to be somewhat guarded and defensive across a broad range of situations. However, situational factors are also important determinants of how an individual will respond in a given situation. Even a person who is usually very trusting of others can become defensive under certain conditions.

The way in which a health care professional speaks to a patient—what is said and the manner in which it is said—will determine, to a great extent, how much trust the patient places in the professional. Good communication builds trust, and trust facilitates open, effective communication.

What do we mean by *trust*? Although we use the word frequently in everyday speech, we seldom bother to define it. Like communication, trust is a complex concept and thus one that is difficult to define precisely. Essentially, trust involves the belief that, in a risky situation, another person will behave toward us in a beneficial way rather than in a harmful way.

The patient who trusts the health professional to act benevolently toward him believes that the professional will recognize and respect the patient's psychological as well as physical vulnerability. This belief enables the patient to discuss his problems and personal concerns openly and honestly, without fear of rejection or ridicule. Under these circumstances, the patient tends to be receptive to new information and more open to the possibility of change.

The patient who does not trust the provider, on the other hand, will behave quite differently. Defensive feelings, which occur when one perceives another person as a potential threat to one's well-being, lead to guarded, self-protective behavior. The patient who feels threatened and defensive will be reluctant to provide much information, especially of a personal nature. Defensiveness also results in closed-mindedness. The defensive patient will not be receptive to new information, nor will he be likely to consider changing his attitudes or behavior. Instead, he is likely to show rigid adherence to his present beliefs and behavior patterns.

There are, unfortunately, many aspects of the dental setting and dental treatment itself that tend to elicit defensiveness in patients. The dental operatory is, after all, a threatening environment. Not only does the patient face the prospect of discomfort and even some pain, but as soon as he opens his mouth, he also exposes himself to the risk of negative, critical comments concerning his oral health status and oral health behavior. For many patients, in fact, this aspect of the dental visit is the most threatening; for some, it is even more threatening than the anesthetic injection or the sound of the handpiece. Results of one survey revealed that the most common cause of patient anxiety and apprehension was "lest the dentist should adopt a negative attitude because of neglect of the teeth." [3] Another researcher asked fearful and nonfearful dental patients to rank 25 factors associated with the dental situation in terms of the anxiety they elicited. The item *dentist tells you that you have bad teeth* was ranked third, while *dentist laughs as he looks in your mouth* was ranked seventh overall. [4]

That the evaluative aspect of dentistry is, for many patients, a particularly aversive feature of the dental visit is not surprising when we consider that, in general, evaluative or judgmental messages—especially if they are strongly negative—are vere likely to stimulate feelings of defensiveness in the receiver. [5] Evaluative messages are those that suggest that the sender has made a judgment of some sort about the other person or about his behavior, beliefs, or attitudes. Examples of negative evaluative statements include the following:

> Your mouth is in bad shape.
> You should have come in a long time ago.
> You haven't been brushing and flossing the way we showed you.
> You've just got to start taking better care of your mouth or you're going to have some real problems.

Messages such as these are apt to elicit defensive feelings in even the most trusting patient. Although your role demands that you evaluate each patient's oral condition and, further, that you share this information with the patient, it is possible to do so in a manner that is less blunt and threatening to the patient's self-esteem. A tactful style of speaking is vital in the dental setting, because even a question as seemingly innocent as "When did you last visit a dentist?" can arouse guilt and anxiety in patients who have not obtained care on a regular basis.

(To obtain this information without evoking guilt, one experienced endodontist suggests asking instead, "What did you have done at your last dental visit?" After the patient replies, you can ask, "And when was that?")[6]

Below are some guidelines to help you avoid or minimize listener defensiveness.

Stress the positive aspects of the patient's oral health status and oral health care behavior. Admittedly, this can be a difficult task with some patients whose mouths reflect serious neglect. Even with patients like these, however, you can at least praise the patient's decision to come in for treatment, even if it is obvious that the decision was postponed well past the point of good sense. When you say, "I'm really glad you came in today," you imply, "You made an intelligent decision." On the other hand, if you say, "If you hadn't waited so long, we wouldn't have so much to do," you are clearly telling the patient, "You behaved stupidly." Which statement is less likely to result in patient defensiveness?

Even when the patient sheepishly points out that he should have come in months or perhaps years earlier, it is not necessary for you to acknowledge this fact; the patient is, after all, well aware of it. Better to simply smile and say, "Well, I'm glad you're here now," or "You're here now and that's the important thing." These responses sound less judgmental and imply that now is a good time to make a new start.

A word of caution: be judicious in your use of the dangerous little word "but." The beneficial effects of a positive message can quickly evaporate if the positive message is linked to one that implies criticism. Compare the following examples:

Poor: Mrs. Atkins, your periodontal condition is improving, BUT you still have to keep working on it.

Good: Mrs. Atkins, your periodontal condition is improving, AND if you keep up the good work, it will continue to get even better.

Poor: Well, Mr. Spencer, I can see that you're doing better with brushing and flossing, BUT you're still not getting these areas back here.

Good: Well, Mr. Spencer, I can see that you're doing better with brushing and flossing, AND now we need to give some special attention to these areas back here.

Describe the problem without blaming or judging the patient. As communication becomes descriptive rather than judgmental, defensiveness diminishes.[5] When you must discuss a problem, describe what you see, not what you think the patient is or what you think his motives are. Avoid labels like "sloppy," "careless," and "irresponsible."

Judgmental: You've been getting a little careless lately. You're going to have to make more of an effort to keep those teeth clean.

Descriptive: I notice that there is quite a bit of plaque and calculus built up in some areas. Let me show you what I mean.

Judgmental: You can't be very concerned about keeping your teeth. If you were, we would see you more often.

Descriptive: Mr. Price, you've told me that you're worried about losing any more teeth. You know that recall visits are very important: The longer the time between visits, the less chance you have of keeping those teeth.

Emphasize sharing information and ideas instead of simply giving instructions and advice. When a speaker conveys the impression that he is in some way superior to the listener, behaves in a dogmatic fashion, and communicates an intention to change or control some aspect of the listener's behavior, the listener will often become defensive.[5] As a dental professional, it is necessary that you think carefully about how you view your role in relating to your patients. Is your view of yourself, "I am an authority and I will tell you what to do"? Or, do you think of yourself as a consultant, retained by the patient for your special knowledge and skills?

The professional who adopts an authoritarian role sees his or her task as one of dispensing instructions and advice to a passive patient who is expected to comply without questioning or objecting. In contrast, for the professional who assumes the role of a consultant, the task becomes one of exploring a variety of options and alternatives with a patient who is an active, responsible participant in his own health care.

The distinctions between these roles are highlighted by marked differences in speaking styles. The Authority often uses phrases like

I think you should . . .
You really ought . . .
I want you to . . .

The Consultant, on the other hand, is more likely to say

Let's discuss how we might . . .
What do you think about . . .
I'd like to explore some ways to . . .

The Consultant approach is far less likely to provoke defensive responses in patients; in addition, the professional who defines his or her role in this manner will probably experience fewer frustrating interactions with patients than the Authority will encounter. Especially in this day of the educated consumer, professionals must expect patients to question recommendations, medications, and treatment plans. In general, it is unwise to expect patients to follow instructions just because they were issued by an "expert." When the professional's behavior reflects respect for the patient's right to make decisions, the likelihood of a successful outcome is greatly enhanced.

THE DECODING PROCESSES:
LISTENING AND RESPONDING SKILLS

> We have been given two ears and but a single mouth in order that we may hear more and talk less.

This ancient quote, attributed to Zeno of Citium, contains advice that is as valuable today as it was many years ago. Listening allows us time to think, to obtain more information, and to understand the information we receive. Listening more and speaking less also increases the emphasis and value of what we say when we do speak.

Listening is not the simple, passive act many people believe it to be. Listening involves more than just hearing. It includes *interpreting* what is heard, a complex process in which incoming sounds are recognized and associated with prior experiences. When sounds have been recognized and interpreted, the listener must then evaluate the information and, finally, decide how he or she will react to it.

Good listening is a prerequisite to understanding, but most people are inefficient listeners. Research has shown that immediately after listening to a ten-minute oral presentation, the average listener has heard, understood, and retained only about *half* of what was said.[7]

Impediments to Good Listening

There are a variety of common habits and attitudes that can interfere with the ability to listen carefully and accurately. They include the following:

Preparing a response while the other person is speaking. The process of interpersonal communication is, ideally, an exchange system in which the participants take turns giving and receiving information. Most people, though, use the time during which another is speaking to plan and prepare what they will say when it is their turn to speak. Obviously, if your attention is focused on what you will say rather than on what is being said to you, you risk missing or mishearing important information.

Listening only to the content of what is said. Most of us listen only for content—for the "facts" of the message. Health care professionals, who are accustomed to collecting certain types of information in order to formulate a diagnosis and treatment plan, are especially prone to listening only for the facts. But emotions, beliefs, and attitudes are also "facts" and have a profound impact upon the listener's understanding of the situation.

Filtering messages to suit our own needs, beliefs, and attitudes. Wise parents are very careful about responding "Maybe" or "We'll see" to a child's request. As many have learned the hard way, children frequently hear these words as a definite "Yes." Of course, children are not the only ones who filter information to suit their own needs: The hygienist who hears a patient's lackluster, "I'll try to do better" as a sincere commitment to improving home care practices is also filtering and distorting the message.

"Nervous" habits and mannerisms, such as fidgeting, drumming the fingers, or fiddling with an instrument or other object, can also interfere with the ability to listen. These behaviors not only divert a portion of your attention from the speaker, but also distract and annoy the speaker.

How do others rate you as a listener? The Listener Self-Test in Figure 3-1 will help you identify annoying listening habits. With practice,

---

Below are a number of listening habits that most people find distracting and annoying. For each item, decide whether you engage in the habit often, sometimes, or never. Score each "Often" response 2, each "Sometimes" 1, and each "Never" 0. If your score is 10 or greater, your listening skills need attention.

	Often	Sometimes	Never
1. I interrupt others.	——	——	——
2. I don't look at others when they talk.	——	——	——
3. I distract the speaker by playing with objects or fidgeting.	——	——	——
4. I look at my watch while others are talking to me.	——	——	——
5. I don't give others a chance to talk.	——	——	——
6. I ask questions that sound as if I doubt everything the speaker says.	——	——	——
7. I correct others' grammar and facts while they're speaking.	——	——	——
8. I finish others' sentences for them.	——	——	——
9. I give conflicting feedback ("body language" says one thing, words another).	——	——	——
10. I keep a "poker face" so the speaker doesn't know if I'm listening or not.	——	——	——

Figure 3-1 Listener Self-Test

poor listening habits can be corrected, and good listening skills can be acquired.

Improving Listening Skills

Health care professionals sometimes object, "I'm so busy that I just can't take the time to listen to all of my patients and co-workers." Actually, good listening seldom requires the investment of additional time. In fact, listening with full and careful attention can save time, because clear communication leads to fewer misunderstandings and costly mistakes.

Perhaps the most crucial ingredient in good listening is putting forth the effort to understand a situation from the other person's point of view. Taking another's perspective requires that we put aside, temporarily, our own view of the situation and that we attempt to see things through the other person's eyes. This task is not as easy as it might seem, because most of us tend to consider our own perspective as the only "reasonable" or "right" way in which to view a situation. It is difficult to remember not only that the other person is likely to view a situation differently from the way we do, but that he has a *right* to have feelings and perceptions that differ from our own. Indeed, it is inevitable that each individual will have his own perception of a situation or event. After all, each of us has a unique genetic inheritance, and we each have our own learning history—a history of failures and successes, joys and sorrows. Each of us, too, has a different assortment of abilities and disabilities, likes and dislikes. All of these factors interact in a very complex fashion to determine how an individual perceives and responds to a particular situation. With this incredible diversity, it is not surprising that individual perceptions differ; rather, the surprising thing is that they are ever similar.

Role playing is an especially useful method for improving your ability to take the other's perspective. Role playing assignments, in which students assume different roles, are worthwhile classroom exercises. If opportunities for formal role playing are not available, you can practice by using interpersonal interactions that occur in your daily life. Try to put yourself in the other person's shoes by asking yourself the following kinds of questions:

How does this situation look to the other person?

How does he or she see me right now?

What aspects of my behavior is the other person responding to?

What events in the other person's recent or distant past might affect his or her interpretation of this situation?

With practice, it is possible to improve your perspective-taking ability and, with it, your ability to communicate effectively with others.

Another listening skill that can be acquired with practice is the art of listening "between the lines" or "below the surface." In social conversation, we usually focus on what is said—the content. We tend to ignore *how* it is said. We become preoccupied with the content of a message and overlook the important feelings and emotions that underlie or accompany the message. Vocal pitch, rate of speech, and speech volume can all serve as indicators of the speaker's emotional state. The sensitive listener uses other cues, too, such as posture and facial expressions, to identify feelings and meanings that are not expressed explicitly. We will discuss nonverbal elements of communication in greater detail later.

Responding and Feedback

Listening involves more than receiving and understanding a message. Effective listening also includes letting the other person know that his message has been received and understood. The good listener communicates attention and interest, as well as understanding of what the speaker has said.

Feedback has a powerful effect on communication and on communicators. A silent, poker-faced listener conveys an impression of being bored or disapproving, which is usually an effective means of silencing the other person and cutting off further communication. *Following* behavior, on the other hand, indicates interest and encourages the speaker to continue to communicate freely. Following behavior includes nonverbal activities such as nodding the head and using facial expressions to convey appropriate emotional responses. Verbal following involves using phrases that express attention and interest, such as "Really?," "Uh-huh," and "I see."

Summarizing and paraphrasing what the speaker has said lets the speaker know that the message has been heard and understood. The following example illustrates the use of summary statements expressed in the listener's own words.

> *Patient*: I was afraid I was going to be late for my appointment this morning. The traffic was just awful. Then I couldn't find a parking place and had to walk four blocks in the rain.
>
> *Dental Professional*: Everything's gone wrong for you this morning.

The most powerful and direct means of communicating understanding is by *active listening*. This style of responding was developed for use in psychotherapy to communicate the therapist's nonjudgmental understanding of the patient's feelings, emotions, and attitudes. The use of this method is not restricted to psychotherapy, however; the same interpersonal factors that are effective in counseling and psychotherapy are also significant in other settings, including industry, education, medicine, nursing, dentistry, and dental hygiene.

Active listening is similar to summarizing and paraphrasing, except that the focus is on the feelings and emotions the speaker expresses—implicitly or explicitly—rather than on the simple content of the message. Compare the following examples:

New Patient: I wasn't really happy with my last dentist. I guess his work was okay, but he wasn't very pleasant. He was always in a rush—never took the time to explain anything. And once, when my little boy got scared when he saw the needle, he told him, "Stop being such a sissy!"

Summary of Content
Dental Professional: You had a bad experience with your last dentist.

Focus on Feelings
Dental Professional: Your experiences with your last dentist have made you a little apprehensive. You wonder how we will treat you here.

Although feelings are not intrinsically more important than content, there are many situations in which focusing on feelings rather than content can clarify and facilitate communication. A response that emphasizes the speaker's feelings indicates that you understand not only the situation, but also the speaker's feelings about the situation. Showing that you have made an effort to view events from the speaker's perspective conveys interest and concern for that person as an individual.

Responses that show acceptance and understanding of feelings are especially useful when you are dealing with a person who is emotionally aroused or upset. Think back to the last time you were angry or worried or frightened. How did others respond to you? Did it help to have another person

offer advice? ("Well, I would just tell him that I wouldn't work one minute past five o'clock and that's that.")

argue with you? ("Oh, I'm sure he didn't mean it that way. He's such a nice person—he'd never do anything like that.")

tell you to calm down? ("Come on, it's silly to be that angry about such a little thing. Getting all excited isn't going to help, you know.")

try to reassure you? ("Don't worry so much about it. It will all blow over and everything will be fine.")

In each case the response was meant to be helpful. But was it? Probably not, because responses such as these amount to little more than arguments or subtle "put-downs." Giving off-the-cuff advice, for example, is really just another way of saying, "I am much wiser than you are, so I will tell you what to do." Nor is arguing about facts and details likely to be helpful to someone who is upset. Even if you believe that the other person is misinformed or mistaken, it is unwise to begin by arguing; by doing so, you immediately place yourself and the other at odds.

The unwary health care professional can easily stumble into the trap of trying to reassure a frightened or worried patient by minimizing or dismissing the feelings he expresses. Telling a patient, "There's nothing to worry about," or "Everything will be just fine," does not really reassure him. Instead, it amounts to telling him that his problem doesn't exist or that he is silly to be concerned about it. When this happens, the patient is hardly likely to perceive the health professional as an understanding or caring person.

As you read the following examples, try to put yourself in the patient's position. Which responses convey awareness and acceptance of the patient's feelings? Which encourage the patient to continue to communicate openly with the dental professional?

Example A

Patient: I get so tense when I have to have dental work done. Sometimes I feel like I could just scream.
Dental Professional: Surely it isn't that bad, now.

The patient has just stated that it is, indeed, "that bad." Contradicting her will not alter her feelings—but she probably won't confide in this dental professional again.

Dental Professional: It must be quite an ordeal for you when you feel so tense and nervous.

This response acknowledges the patient's feelings and encourages continued communication.

Example B

Patient: I almost fainted when Dr. Wilson told me how much my treatment would cost. It's just outrageous! Why, I could buy a new car for that kind of money.
Dental Professional: Yes, but a new car will wear out in a few years. Good dental work will last much longer.

This response ignores the patient's feelings and amounts to little more than arguing with the patient. A patient who is upset is seldom receptive to a lecture.

> *Dental Professional*: It's upsetting to find out that your dental work will cost more than you expected—especially when there are other things you would like to do with the money.

This response acknowledges the patient's feelings of shock and dismay without, however, indicating agreement that the fees are "outrageous."

Johnson offers these general guidelines for using active listening to communicate accurate understanding:

1. Restate the sender's expressed feelings and meanings in your own words. Do not mimic or parrot the speaker's exact words.
2. Preface your responses with "You feel . . . ," "It seems to you . . . ," "You mean . . ." and so on.
3. Avoid any indication of approval or disapproval, agreement or disagreement. Your response must be nonevaluative.
4. Make your nonverbal messages consistent with your verbal messages. Look attentive, interested, open to the other person's ideas and feelings.[7]

Although active listening appears easy, considerable practice is required to use this style of responding comfortably and with skill. How can you obtain this practice? Johnson suggests:

> Follow this rule the next time you get deeply involved in a conversation or argument: *Each person can speak up for himself only after he has first restated the ideas and feelings of the previous sender accurately and to the sender's satisfaction.* This means that, before presenting your own point of view, it would be necessary for you to achieve the other's frame of reference, to understand his thoughts and feelings so well that you could paraphrase them for him. Sounds simple? Try it; you will find that it is one of the most difficult things you have ever attempted. You will also find that your arguments will become much more constructive and productive if you are able to follow the above rule successfully.[7]

REFERENCES

1. Howard, W.W. *Dental practice planning.* St. Louis: C.V. Mosby, 1975.
2. Jan, H.W. General semantic orientation in dentist-patient relations. *Journal of the American Dental Association* 68:424, 1964.

3. Forsberg, A. Odontologiska faculteten vid Karolinska institutet. *Sven Tandlak Tidskr* 59:147, 1966.

4. Gale, E. Fears of the dental situation. *Journal of Dental Research* 51:964, 1972.

5. Gibb, J.R. Defensive communication. *Journal of Communication* 11:141, 1961.

6. McDonnell, C. Personal communication, April, 1982.

7. Johnson, D.W., and Matross, R.P. Attitude modification methods. In *Helping people change*, edited by F. Kanfer and A. Goldstein. New York: Pergamon Press, 1975.

4

Nonverbal Communication

For most people, the term *nonverbal communication* is virtually synonymous with the expression *body language.* But while body posture, gestures, and facial expressions can and do convey very important information, nonverbal communication, in the fullest sense, involves much more.

When we speak of nonverbal communication, we are referring to a multiplicity of cues which, by design or unintentionally, convey messages to those around us. Nonverbal cues range from the very subtle—a tiny flicker of surprise or fear, an all-but-imperceptible wince—to the most obvious: The message implicit in a snarling facial expression and a raised, clenched fist is clear in any language. Nor do we convey nonverbal messages only through our moment-to-moment behavior: The arrangement and decoration of the environment in which we place ourselves, and the way in which we clothe, adorn, and groom our bodies make definite statements about how we see ourselves, who we are, and what we do.

Nonverbal messages can be deliberate and intentional, like the frown and shake of the head that signal "Stop that!" or "That's wrong." Often, though, nonverbal communication is unintentional and occurs without the sender's awareness. A person who feels impatient or annoyed, for example, might drum his fingers or tap his toes without really being aware of these behaviors. Similarly, a person who is anxious might nervously chew on his lip or fingernails.

Nonverbal signals and cues serve many important purposes in communication. For example, communication researchers have discovered that in the average conversation between two people, the verbal components carry less than 35 percent of the social meaning of the situation, while more than 65 percent is conveyed through nonverbal messages.[1] Nonverbal behavior is especially important in communicating feelings, emotions, and liking or disliking: It has been estimated that, of the total liking or affection we communicate to another person, only 7 percent is communicated through words.[2] Voice cues, such as pitch and volume, carry 38 percent of the liking communicated, and facial expression and gaze communicate 55 percent.

As important as nonverbal communication is in other settings, there is reason to believe that nonverbal behavior is particularly crucial in the dental setting. Because anxiety is usually accompanied by increased vigilance and scanning of the social and physical environment, dental patients are likely to be especially observant of and sensitive to the dental professional's nonverbal behavior. If your verbal messages are congruent with your nonverbal messages, and both convey competence and concern and caring for the patient, then the patient can relax and trust you. If, on the other hand, the patient detects inconsistencies and contradictions between your verbal and nonverbal messages, he is apt to respond with apprehensiveness and mistrust. Clearly, then, it is to your advantage to pay careful attention to the nonverbal aspects of your communication.

In turn, of course, much valuable information can be gained by learning to attend closely to your patients' nonverbal behavior. As we might expect, health care professionals who are sensitive to their patients' nonverbal cues are better able to establish good rapport with them. Research has shown, for example, that physicians who are more skilled at observing and understanding nonverbal communication meet with greater success in terms of patient satisfaction.[3]

There are a number of widely held myths concerning nonverbal behavior. Many recent books and articles have popularized the notion that all nonverbal behavior carries a specific message. A related belief is that if one is sufficiently skilled at detecting and interpreting these messages, one can practically read another person's mind. These notions have been referred to as "myths" by specialists who study communication because, as they point out, no single gesture, movement, or facial expression has only a single, unvarying meaning. Shaking the head slowly from side to side, for instance, can mean "No," "I don't know," or "That's unbelievable." Because a single bit of nonverbal behavior does not occur in isolation, apart from the context in which it occurs, it cannot be interpreted in isolation. The significance of a piece of nonverbal behavior depends on many complex factors, such as the verbal and nonverbal behaviors that accompany it and those that have preceded it during the particular interaction. If, for example, you saw a man place his hand over his heart while talking with another man, you would need more information in order to distinguish whether he was gesturing "On my word of honor" or talking about his recent heart attack.

THE FUNCTIONS OF NONVERBAL BEHAVIOR

Nonverbal behavior serves a variety of communicative functions. An awareness of the ways in which nonverbal behavior is commonly used can help you become more sensitive to your own nonverbal behavior and to that of others.

Substitution

Nonverbal messages can substitute for verbal messages: A nod indicates wordless agreement, a shake of the head signals disagreement, and a wave can take the place of the words *hello* or *goodbye.* Nonverbal substitutes are often quite obvious and present no problem to the person who must interpret them; a hand placed briefly over an empty cup says "No refills, thanks" to hosts and waiters in virtually all corners of the globe. But problems can arise when nonverbal signals and messages are not so immediately obvious to the receiver, especially if the sender believes that his nonverbal cues are clear and easy to interpret. If you fail to recognize, from his posture and facial expression, that a coworker is depressed or upset, you might be seen as indifferent or uncaring. If you are often on the receiving end of such complaints as, "You should have known that I was upset!" and "Couldn't you tell that I was angry?" you would be well-advised to pay closer attention to the nonverbal behavior of those around you.

On the other hand, it isn't a good idea to rely excessively on nonverbal behavior to signal your own emotional state, your preferences, and your current state of mind to others. An adolescent, who has not yet mastered more direct forms of communicating, might slam doors to announce that he is angry or gaze mournfully out a window to indicate that he is troubled or unhappy. Adults are expected to communicate more directly. Simple statements like, "I'm a little out of sorts today," or "I'm feeling pretty low" can help to avoid misunderstandings and hurt feelings.

Enhancement

Nonverbal messages are often used to confirm and enhance verbal messages. Examples include pounding a table top while exclaiming, "I'm so angry!" or beaming and patting someone's shoulder while saying, "Nice job. I'm really proud of you." When used in this way, nonverbal behavior emphasizes and repeats verbal behavior, which helps to ensure that the listener grasps the speaker's point.

Nonverbal behavior also adds color, drama, and depth to communication. When nonverbal messages are used to complement verbal messages, another dimension is added to communication, just as the use of stereo equipment enhances the experience of listening to music.

An especially important point for health care professionals to remember is that when nonverbal messages echo verbal messages, the patient feels secure in trusting the professional. Writing from the perspective of one who has studied the subject intensively, Howard Friedman has observed that "one of the most critical aspects of effective treatment involves neither just what is said nor just how it is said. Rather, what is often more important is the degree of consistency between verbal and nonverbal cues." When there are inconsistencies between verbal and nonverbal messages, the professional is likely to be perceived as insincere and, therefore, untrustworthy.[4] For example, if a positive statement such as "It's nice to see you" is accompanied by a facial expression that indicates some anger, the speaker might be seen as sarcastic or nasty. The same verbal statement accompanied by a sad facial expression might convey indifference.

Contradiction

Nonverbal messages can, in some instances, confuse or contradict the verbal message, as when the phrase, "Oh, I'd just love to do that!" is said with a grimace and a sarcastic inflection. If this is done intentionally to convey sarcasm, it can add humor and variety to communication. (Of course, it is important to remember that a little sarcasm goes a long way in most interactions. People who use sarcasm excessively are often perceived by others as aloof, critical, and cold. Sarcasm should be used sparingly, if at all, in the dental setting.)

Contradictions and inconsistencies between verbal and nonverbal behavior sometimes occur unintentionally, without the sender's awareness. Even when they are not deliberate, discrepancies between verbal and nonverbal messages can result in feelings of mistrust, distress, and dislike for the communicator.

Regulating

Finally, nonverbal behaviors are used to regulate the flow of communication between participants. Nonverbal cues can function like traffic signals to regulate conversational beginnings and endings, turn-taking in conversation, and changes in subject. For example, when you finish an utterance and expect your listener to start talking, your voice will probably drop slightly in volume, you will increase eye contact with the listener, and your body will become slightly more relaxed. These cues signal the other person, "I'm finished; go ahead." If the listener neither begins to speak nor signals you nonverbally to continue, you might send more obvious signals such as raising your eyebrows as if to say "Well?"

Other nonverbal behaviors are used to signal a request for a speaking turn. Opening the mouth while inhaling, nodding the head rapidly, and holding an index finger upraised all indicate, "I have something to say now."

Leave-taking situations typically involve a great deal of nonverbal signals. Two of the most frequently observed are decreased eye gaze and positioning of the body toward the exit. Other leave-taking behaviors include looking at one's watch, rapid head-nodding, and, if seated, placing hands on thighs for leverage in getting out of a chair.

In driving an automobile, a driver who ignores traffic signals would be considered a very poor driver—"unsafe at any speed." So, too, the person who ignores nonverbal regulatory cues is apt to be perceived as a poor communicator. The listener who frequently interrupts before the speaker has finished is seen as rude; the speaker who consistently refuses to yield a speaking turn is viewed as selfish and domineering; and the listener who often fails to respond to signals that it is his turn to speak will be thought inattentive.

FORMS OF NONVERBAL COMMUNICATION

Nonverbal communication, as we have mentioned, takes many forms, including posture, body movements, and gestures; facial expressions and eye contact; tactile, or touching, behavior; use of space, distance, and time; and paralinguistic cues—vocal cues such as rate, tone, and pitch.

Posture, Body Movement, and Gestures

As is the case with nonverbal behavior in general, communication researchers often classify gestures and body movements according to the communicative functions served. *Emblems*, for example, are gestures or movements that have direct verbal translations, such as the "A-OK" sign which means "Everything is fine," or bringing the hand up to the mouth to symbolize eating. Emblems are used to substitute for words, especially when verbal communication is difficult or impossible.

Unlike emblems, which are used instead of words, *illustrators* accompany speech. Illustrators accentuate what is said verbally, such as spreading the arms wide while verbally describing great size.

Gestures and body movements often serve as *regulators.* As we have discussed, these signals function to regulate the flow of communication.

Finally, *adaptors* are the unconscious movements often associated with boredom, anxiety, or impatience. Adaptors include such "nervous mannerisms" as tapping the fingers or toes, fidgeting, and picking at or rubbing parts of the body.

Posture and body movements are especially important in conveying attitudes of liking and warmth and, conversely, dislike and coldness. Nonverbal cues associated with warmth and liking include a relaxed but alert posture, leaning forward of the body toward the other person, direct eye contact, and hands relaxed and still. On the other hand, slumping or leaning away from the other person, or gazing at the ceiling and drumming the fingers signal coldness and dislike.

When these behaviors have been examined in health care settings, the findings have been consistent with those obtained in other settings.[5] Patient satisfaction with the health care professional is greater when the professional faces the patient, leans forward, with chin in hands, and gazes directly at the patient. Patient satisfaction is less with a professional who leans back, with elevated chin, and gazes over the patient's head. Further, patients understand and remember more of what they are told by a "warm" professional than by a professional whose nonverbal behaviors signal "cold."

Body posture and gestures are also important clues to lying and deception. Most people are fairly skilled at controlling their facial expressions when attempting to deceive another person but tend to forget about controlling other parts of the body. Thus, the deceiver might tap his feet or change leg position frequently. Hands, too, can "leak" information.

The task of observing and interpreting a dental patient's nonverbal behavior is made more difficult by the fact that these cues are often quite subtle. As researchers Kleinknecht and Bernstein have reported, very few anxious adults exhibit such obvious signs of fear as trembling visibly or clutching the arms of the dental chair.[6] Of course, this is not to say that anxious patients give *no* nonverbal clues to their feelings. The signals are usually subtle, however, and probably consist of fleeting changes in facial expression and small, quick eye movements, rather than of more easily detected gestures or movements.

Facial Expression and Eye Contact

The face, with its many fine muscles and complex innervation, is a principal source of nonverbal communication. Facial expressions carry more detailed and specific information than is conveyed through other nonverbal channels. The facial expressions associated with the six so-called primary emotions—surprise, fear, anger, happiness, sorrow, and disgust—seem to be universally recognized across all cultures.[7]

An interest in, and responsiveness to, the human face appears to be "programmed" into the human infant from birth. When newborns are shown designs that resemble the human face, they follow the designs with their eyes. Much less visual following occurs with designs that do not resemble a human face.[8]

At about one year of age, children are able to recognize some distinct facial expressions; as children mature, they learn to identify more subtle and complex facial expressions. With increasing age, children also learn to control their own facial expressions. Not only do they master the ability to use facial expressions to convey what they feel, but they also learn when and where certain expressions are considered appropriate. Most of this learning occurs through observation of others, but some direct teaching can occur, as when a parent or teacher says, "Wipe that smile off your face," or "Don't you dare look at me like that!"

Just as we learn how to reveal our emotions through our facial expressions, we also learn to conceal emotions that we do not wish others to observe. We learn, for example, to hide unhappiness or disappointment under a smile and to cover feelings of anger, annoyance, or disgust beneath a bland expression. In fact, as we noted in the preceding section, most people are fairly adept at controlling their facial expressions. For this reason, the face is usually a poor source of clues for detecting attempts to deceive.

Which part of the face best reveals emotions? According to Mark Knapp, widely recognized scholar in the field of nonverbal communication, no one area of the face is "best." Instead,

For any given emotion, a particular area of the face may carry the most important information for identification. For disgust the nose/cheek/mouth area is crucial; for fear it is the eyes/eyelids; for sadness we would do well to examine the brows/forehead and eyes/eyelids; the important areas for happiness seem to be the cheeks/mouth and brows/forehead areas; and surprise can be seen in any of the three areas of the face.[9]

In a previous section, we discussed the importance of providing feedback to let the other person know that you are listening with interest and attention. The face is a major source of such feedback. A good listener's facial expression reflects some of the emotion the speaker is describing—a sad look when an unhappy event is recounted; an excited, anticipatory expression when the speaker is describing a pleasant surprise. By using facial expressions to "mirror" another's emotions, we indicate unmistakably that we are involved in what he is saying.

The eye region is a major source of information in facial expression. The significance of the eyes in human interaction is reflected in the great number of phrases and sayings about eyes and eye behavior. Some familiar examples are, "The eyes are the windows of the soul," "the evil eye," "if looks could kill," and "wide-eyed innocence."

Eye contact and gaze play a powerful role in the initiation and development of interpersonal relationships from the earliest moments of human life. We know that human infants can see at birth,[10] and it has been suggested that the tendency of the newborn to focus on the eyes of persons holding them serves to elicit innate mothering responses from adults.[11] Certainly, mothers of newborns are eager to make eye-to-eye contact with their babies. When this is not possible (as in the case of blind infants), mothers have difficulty in feeling close to their babies: "Without the affirmation of mutual gazing, mothers feel lost and like strangers to their babies until both learn to substitute other means of communication."[12]

In any situation, eye behavior is influenced by such factors as the relationship between the participants, the physical distance between them, and the topics under discussion. In an interaction between two people who differ in status, for example, the lower-status person will tend to gaze more at the higher-status person than the reverse. Physical distance increases the amount of eye contact, while close proximity leads to a decrease, especially if the people involved are strangers. We obtain a certain amount of psychological privacy in a crowded elevator by carefully avoiding eye contact with others. Many dental patients obtain this privacy by simply closing their eyes during treatment.

Eye contact is commonly associated with interest and attention: The phrase "all eyes" denotes rapt attention. Conversely, lack of eye contact is usually interpreted as lack of interest, concern, or caring. Sometimes, too, failure to meet another's eyes is associated with guilt or attempts to deceive.

Of course, it is not advisable to stare at the person with whom you are speaking during every second of an interaction. To do so would, as you can imagine, produce discomfort and anxiety. A "normal" amount of gazing has been estimated as slightly less than half of the time during which you are the speaker and about three-quarters of the time during which you are the listener.[13]

Touch

From infancy, touch plays a crucial role in psychological and social development. Over two decades ago, Harlow's famous studies of young monkeys raised with surrogate mothers made of wire and cloth demonstrated the importance of physical contact for normal primate development. More recently, research on mother-infant interaction has supported the idea that touch is also essential for healthy development among humans.

The symbolic role of touch has a long history in the healing arts. In the Middle Ages, many people believed that the king's touch had curative powers. Even today, faith healers use "laying on of hands" to restore believers to health. Some writers have made the blanket assumption that, in health care settings, touch is always reassuring and beneficial to the patient. One writer states that "in nursing, touch may be the most important of all nonverbal behaviors." [14] Another writer goes even further: Touch "should be considered an indispensable part of the doctor's art" and "always enhances . . . therapeutic abilities." [15]

We might well ask whether such statements are supported by research evidence. Unfortunately, there appears to be no research on this subject in the dental literature, and studies in medical settings have produced confusing results. While one study found that touch behavior by nurses improved patients' attitudes toward nurses,[16] another study showed that physician touch during the first visit was actually associated with *lower* levels of patient satisfaction with the physician.[5]

How can we explain these discrepancies? We must remember that touching, like any other behavior, does not occur in isolation. Rather, touching is just a single element in an interpersonal interaction that is likely to consist of many factors, interrelated in a complex fashion. The setting in which touching occurs is important, and so are the patterns of verbal and nonverbal behavior that precede, accompany, and follow a touch, and the personal histories of each of the participants. Some people enjoy touching and being touched. Other people, probably as a result of many earlier experiences, find physical contact with others uncomfortable.

Unfortunately, then, we can offer few general rules, other than those dictated by sensitivity and good sense. The following are some guidelines to keep in mind:

Children generally find gentle physical contact, such as touching, patting, or stroking, comforting and soothing. Touch is also a useful way to prompt desired behavior in young children. A directive such as "Hands in your lap" is both more pleasant and more effective if accompanied by gentle physical guidance and a little pat when the hands are in place.

A touch on the hand, arm, or shoulder can be reassuring to a patient who is obviously anxious or in pain. Note, however, that there is a difference between a light, compassionate touch that says, "I'm concerned about you" and the brisker sort of pat that implies a condescending, "There, there—nothing to fuss about." The difference is subtle but, to the patient, very real.

Space and Time

In his popular book, *The Territorial Imperative*, Robert Ardrey argues that all animals, including man, engage in territorial behavior; that is, they lay claim to territory around themselves and defend this area against invaders. Territory, in this sense, refers not only to a specific geographic spot, but to the area of personal space immediately surrounding an individual.

The rules governing the ways in which members of a particular culture use space are seldom, if ever, explicitly taught. Parents do not say to their children, "Now, remember: Stand this close to a friend and only this close to your teacher." Nor, for the most part, are we consciously aware of observing these rules. But the existence of these unspoken norms quickly becomes apparent if they are violated. When personal space is invaded, people react with discomfort, anxiety, and annoyance. We fidget uneasily, for example, if someone stands too close in an empty elevator or if another person spreads his books and papers on "our" side of the library table. In the latter case, it is likely that the person whose territory has been invaded will get up and move to another table. If escape is not possible, annoyance sometimes becomes anger, or even aggression; the all-too-common highway practice of tailgating is an example of space violation that is likely to be met with angry shouts and rude gestures from the victim.

Rules concerning personal distance vary from culture to culture. You can probably appreciate this if you have ever had the experience of conversing with someone from a Latin American country. Because Latin Americans tend to stand closer to each other than North Americans usually do, you might have felt crowded and have spent much of the conversation backing away.

Norms also vary within a culture, depending on such factors as the age, sex, and relative status of the participants in an interaction. For instance, women stand closer together than men do, and children closer than adults. The nature of the interaction and the relationship between the participants are also important determinants of distance. Acquaintances sit or stand closer to each other than strangers do, and friends closer than acquaintances. Conversational distance is also influenced by whether the topic is pleasant or unpleasant.

Anthropologist Edward T. Hall has identified distinct zones in which social interactions occur in our culture.[17] These zones range in distance from what Hall calls the "public zone," the distance used for public lectures and speeches, to the "intimate zone," which ranges from a distance of about 18 inches to actual physical contact. The intimate zone is usually reserved for interactions between lovers, spouses, and parents and children.

Dental treatment is one of the exceptions to this rule. In order to provide treatment, the dental professional must invade the patient's intimate zone. While this invasion is unavoidable, it is important to remember that it can induce considerable discomfort in many patients. In discussing this dilemma, one writer suggests that you try to give the patient "breathing room" when possible.[18] After you complete a procedure, move away from the patient for a moment to allow a bit of spatial privacy.

We should note that it is not only the patient who experiences discomfort related to the close proximity necessary during dental treatment. A colleague addressing a group of dental hygienists on the topic of nonverbal behavior in the dental operatory was surprised at the number of questions and comments from the audience concerning flirtatious behavior from opposite-sex patients during and after dental treatment. Nurses, who often must enter the patient's personal space, also report encountering this sort of situation with some frequency.[19] Some patients, taught from childhood to associate physical closeness with personal intimacy, apparently have difficulty separating the two.

This situation, obviously, can be very awkward, so it is probably worthwhile to take preventive measures. Does this mean that you must be aloof and very formal with all opposite-sex patients? Not at all, but it is quite possible to show warmth and concern while maintaining a professional demeanor. It is a good idea, for example, to avoid bantering and teasing with opposite-sex patients, especially those you don't know very well. This behavior is often perceived as flirtatious and, while appropriate and enjoyable in many social settings, really has no place in a professional setting. Remember, too, that use of first names suggests a social relationship rather than a professional one. Uniforms also help to signal that this is a professional interaction rather than a social relationship.

Like personal space, time is an important but seldom recognized aspect of interpersonal communication. As a professional to whom "time is money," you share the belief common to people in North American and Northern European countries that time is naturally fixed into seconds, minutes, hours, days of the week, and so on. We take for granted that time can be segmented and scheduled, saying "This will only take about an hour," "The train leaves at six," and "I'll see you at one-thirty."

We sometimes forget that members of other cultures do not always share our concept of time. Americans who go abroad to such countries as Iran and Afghanistan are often frustrated by the differences in the way time is handled. Even within the borders of the United States, there can be marked differences. Hall[17] notes, for example, that the Sioux Indians have no word for *waiting* or *late*.[17] This reflects the fact that, to the Indians, time meant a natural succession of days beginning with the new moon and ending with the old. The practice of dividing time into strange and unnatural periods such as hours and minutes was difficult for them to comprehend and has resulted in many misunderstandings over the years.

Especially in our time-conscious culture, where promptness is highly valued, it is considered insulting to keep someone waiting. In the dental setting, an additional problem is created when patients are kept waiting: In general, the patient's anxiety increases with the length of the wait. Of course, there are times in even the most efficient practice when a patient must be kept waiting. When a delay is unavoidable, courtesy dictates that the patient be given an apology, as well as an explanation. Most people will tolerate a wait with good grace if they understand that Dr. Jones is treating an emergency patient. Without an explanation, however, patients are apt to imagine Dr. Jones chatting with a stock broker or setting up a golf date, and patience can quickly wear thin.

Remember, too, not to leave a patient unattended in the chair for longer than the briefest possible time. If you must leave the patient for a more extended period, explain your absence, put the chair in an upright position, and offer to bring the patient a magazine. Your patients will appreciate this attention and courtesy.

IMPROVING NONVERBAL AWARENESS

The late Milton Erickson, who has often been called the father of clinical hypnosis, placed strong emphasis on the importance of observing a patient's nonverbal behavior. His own powers of observation and skill in nonverbal communication were legendary. On one occasion, for example, Dr. Erickson astonished a professional audience by hypnotizing a woman using only nonverbal signals. Verbal communication between Dr. Erickson and the woman was impossible, because she spoke only Spanish and he spoke only English.[20]

On another occasion, while speaking before a large audience,

Dr. Erickson paused for a moment and, saying nothing of what he was doing, secretly wrote down a prediction. The prediction was that at a certain point in his talk, two people from the audience—both strangers to Dr. Erickson—would come down to the podium and sit beside him. This would occur without any apparent instruction from him. Erickson not only predicted who the people would be, he also predicted who would take the chair on his left and who the chair on his right. When he reached the point in his lecture, known only to him, the audience was startled to see two women arise from their seats, walk slowly down the aisle, and seat themselves beside Dr. Erickson, each in the chair he had predicted she would select.[21]

How did Dr. Erickson perform this feat? Early in his lecture he had observed that both women looked very attentive and seemed absorbed in what he was saying. From long experience, he knew that this *response attentiveness* meant that a person would be especially receptive to suggestion. As he lectured, Dr. Erickson repeated numerous nonverbal signals, accompanied by subtle verbal cues, to suggest the desired behavior to the women. For example, while apparently letting his eyes roam around the audience at random, he let his gaze linger on each woman just as he said something like, "As suggestions are given, *you* . . . ," and "When *you* are ready. . . ." These suggestions were very subtle and were incorporated into the lecture in such a manner that no one, including the women, was aware of Erickson's intent. When Erickson saw certain facial and postural cues indicating that all was ready, he simply said, "Now that you are ready . . . walk down and take your proper seats." The women responded as he had intended they would.

Milton Erickson obviously was not born with such remarkable powers. Rather, his great skill developed as a result of his efforts to overcome his own physical handicaps. Born tone-deaf, he learned to pay careful attention to inflections in the voices of others and to make subtle but powerful suggestions through his own use of tone and inflection. Then, at the age of 17, a polio attack left him paralyzed. Of this experience, he reported:

> I lay in bed without a sense of body awareness. . . . I spent hours trying to locate my hand or my foot or my toes by a sense of feeling, so I became acutely aware of what movements were . . . [and] this has been exceedingly useful. People use those little telltale movements, those adjustive movements that are so revealing if one can notice them. So much of our communication is in our bodily movements.[22]

It should not be inferred that practice alone will enable you to match Dr. Erickson's skills; Milton Erickson was unique—many have called him a genius. But learning to observe nonverbal behavior can improve your sensitivity to others and your ability to communicate effectively with them. Structured classroom exercises offer an ideal opportunity not only to hone your ability to detect nonverbal signals sent by others, but also to devote attention to your own nonverbal behavior. If such opportunities are not available to you, your everyday life experiences can offer many excellent opportunities to learn by observing the people around you. You can begin, for example, by observing people in such public places as trains, buses, and waiting rooms. Try to determine whether the person next to you is tense or relaxed, calm or anxious. What nonverbal cues did you use in making your assessment?

When you are in conversation with another person, observe to what degree the other person is absorbed in what you are saying. Is the person leaning forward, body quiet, gaze fixed on your face as you talk? Or do you detect some restless leg or hand movements or a wandering gaze? Then learn to watch for these behaviors in your patients. The patient whose nonverbal behavior indicates that his attention is fixed on what you are saying is far more likely to be open to the changes you suggest than is the patient whose nonverbal behavior suggests boredom or a polite pretense of interest and attention. It is not suggested that you simply give up when faced with the latter sort of patient, but you can save both yourself and the patient considerable frustration by soft-pedaling your efforts, until and unless a better relationship can be established.

REFERENCES

1. McCroskey, J.C., Larson, C.E., and Knapp, M.L. *Introduction to interpersonal communication.* Englewood Cliffs, N.J.: Prentice-Hall, 1971.
2. Mehrabian, A., and Ferris, S.R. Inference of attitudes from nonverbal communication in two channels. *Journal of Consulting Psychology* 31:248, 1967.
3. Di Matteo, M.R., Friedman, H.S., and Taranta, A. Sensitivity to bodily nonverbal communication as a factor in practitioner-patient rapport. *Journal of Nonverbal Behavior* 4:18, 1979.
4. Friedman, H.S. Nonverbal communication between patients and medical practitioners. *Journal of Social Issues* 35:82, 1979.
5. Larsen, K.M., and Smith, C.K. Assessment of nonverbal communication in the patient-physician interview. *Journal of Family Practice* 12:481, 1981.
6. Kleinknecht, R.A., and Bernstein, D.A. The assessment of dental fear. *Behavior Therapy* 9:626, 1978.
7. Eckman, P. Cross-cultural studies of facial expression. In *Darwin and facial expression*, edited by P. Ekman. New York: Academic Press, 1973.
8. Goren, C., Sarty, M., and Wu, P. Visual following and pattern discrimination of face-like stimuli by newborn infants. *Pediatrics* 56:544, 1975.
9. Knapp, M.L. *Essentials of nonverbal communication.* New York: Holt, Rinehart, and Winston, 1980.

10. Brazelton, T.B., School, M.L., and Robey, J.S. Visual responses in the newborn. *Pediatrics* 37:284, 1966.

11. Robson, K.S. The role of eye-to-eye contact in maternal-infant attachment. *Journal of Child Psychology* 8:13, 1967.

12. Klaus, M.H., and Kennell, J.H. *Maternal-infant bonding.* St. Louis: C.V. Mosby, 1976.

13. Argyle, M., and Ingham, R. Gaze, mutual gaze, and proximity. *Semiotica* 6:32, 1972.

14. Blondis, M.N., and Jackson, B.E. *Nonverbal communication with patients.* New York: John Wiley, 1977.

15. Montague, A. *Touching.* New York: Harper and Row, Pub., 1978.

16. Agulera, D.C. Relationship between physical contact and verbal interaction between nurses and patients. *Journal of Psychiatric Nursing* 5:5, 1967.

17. Hall, E.T. *The silent language.* New York: Doubleday, 1959.

18. Kreps, G.L. Nonverbal communication in dentistry. *Dental Assistant* 50:18, 1981.

19. Johnson, B.S. The meaning of touch in nursing. *Nursing Outlook*, 13:59, 1965.

20. Erickson, M.H. Pantomime techniques in hypnosis and the implications. *American Journal of Clinical Hypnosis* 7:64, 1964.

21. Erickson, M.H. The "Surprise" and "My-Friend-John" techniques of hypnosis: Minimal cues and natural field experimentation. *American Journal of Clinical Hypnosis* 6:293, 1964.

22. Haley, J. (ed.) *Advanced techniques of hypnosis and therapy.* New York: Grune and Stratton, 1967.

5

Understanding Dental Fear

The scene: a busy street corner in a medium-size city. A roving reporter, armed with a tape recorder, stops passers-by to ask them, "How do you feel about going to the dentist?" Responses vary. Some smile or laugh; many more grimace and even shudder. Among the replies are the following:

> *Construction Worker, age 35*: I don't much like it, I'll tell you. In fact, I'd have to say that I'd rather be laid up with the flu than to have to go to the dentist.
>
> *Secretary, age 26*: I hate it. I just hate it! If I have a dentist's appointment in the afternoon, I get so worked up I can hardly even go to work in the morning. I get so nervous, I actually feel sick.
>
> *Police Officer, age 43*: The dentist? Well, I'm a little ashamed to admit it, but I haven't been to the dentist since . . . oh, it must be five or six years now. I know I should go; I've got some teeth that are real bad. But when I think about that needle—whew!

THE INCIDENCE AND ETIOLOGY OF DENTAL FEAR

How prevalent are attitudes such as those expressed in the responses above? If we were to interview every man and woman in the United States, we would find many who would express similar sentiments. In fact, it is estimated that as many as twelve million adults describe themselves as highly fearful of dental treatment.[1] Many are so fearful that they avoid dental treatment until pain forces them to seek care. In a recent survey in which respondents were asked their reasons for not seeing a dentist when they felt they should, one-third said that fear was the principal obstacle.[2]

Women tend to report more fear of dentistry than men do, although this might simply reflect the fact that, in our society, it is more acceptable for women to admit feelings of fear and apprehensiveness.

Dental fear is also related to age. Among children, the percentage of those who fear dental treatment appears to be even higher than it is among the adult population. Some have placed the figure as high as 16 percent.[3] While it is common for toddlers and youngsters below the age of three or four years to cry and protest during dental procedures, most children master their fear and are reasonably calm, cooperative patients by the age of five. The elementary-school–age child who continues to show marked fear might not outgrow the fear without special help, but might instead grow up to be a fearful, avoidant adult.

Factors such as income and educational level are associated with fear of dentistry. Studies have shown that people of lower socioeconomic status tend to be more fearful than those from middle and upper socioeconomic groups.[2] Why might this be the case? Among the poor and less-educated members of our society, routine dental care is much less common than it is among the affluent and well-educated. Symptomatically based or emergency visits, more common among lower socioeconomic groups, often result in extensive or painful treatment. (One investigation, for example, revealed that, as income level decreases, the probability that the patient had extractions or oral surgery at his last dental visit increases.[4]) This pattern probably accounts for differences in dental fear between socioeconomic groups.

FEAR: ITS EFFECTS ON PROVIDER AND PATIENT

The Effects of Patient Anxiety on the Provider

Dental professionals readily acknowledge that tense, anxious patients are a source of considerable concern to them. When dentists are asked to list patient-management problems they encounter, fear is the problem cited most frequently.[5] Fear also ranks among the patient-management problems that dentists considered most troublesome.

Apart from humanitarian considerations, there are sound reasons that dental health care providers need to be knowledgeable about the detection and treatment of dental fear. Working long hours in close contact with patients who are tense and anxious can be a significant source of stress for the professional. As we have previously noted, the emotional states of those around us—even of strangers—can quickly influence our own emotional states. Time spent in the company of a person who is relaxed and serene can have a soothing effect, but even a few minutes of interaction with a tense, jittery person can produce unpleasant feelings of tension and arousal. An entire workday spent in such company is likely to exhaust even the most energetic professional.

Besides adversely affecting the health professional's emotional well-being, fearful patients pose many office-management problems. Fear and avoidance are, of course, closely related; fearful patients are three times more likely than nonfearful patients to fail a scheduled appointment.[6] Thus, anxious patients can wreak havoc with a dental schedule.

An anxious patient can also have deleterious effects on efficiency. During tooth preparation, these patients are more likely to interrupt drilling, thereby increasing chair time and decreasing efficiency.[7] In fact, highly anxious patients have been found to require as much as 20 percent more chair time than nonfearful patients, even for routine procedures.

The Effects of Fear on the Patient

The relationship between anxiety and pain.   Many patients who fear dental treatment cite pain as the principal reason for their fear. This can be somewhat puzzling to the dental professional, because, thanks to technological and pharmacological advances, dental treatment is seldom accompanied by severe pain. What is often overlooked, however, is the extent to which pain and anxiety are intertwined.

In the past, theories of pain perception attempted to explain pain solely in terms of neurophysiological events, such as the number of neurons firing and the rate at which they fire. Pain, according to this model, occurs only in response to tissue damage or organic pathology, and the intensity of pain is directly proportional to the amount of damage sustained or noxious stimulation applied.

More recent evidence indicates that pain is *not* simply a sensory experience, nor can it be defined only in terms of physiological events. Consider, for example, the athlete injured in a heated contest or the soldier wounded in combat. Neither may even notice the pain until the game or the battle has ended. On the other hand, pain can occur in the absence of tissue damage or disease, and it can persist long after damaged tissue has healed.

These examples, together with a large body of clinical and laboratory research, indicate the importance of psychological factors in the perception and experience of pain. Among the most important of these factors is anxiety. The evidence points to a direct relationship between anxiety and acute pain: When one is emotionally aroused and believes oneself to be threatened or in danger, pain sensitivity is increased.[8,9] Conversely, methods that reduce anxiety also reduce pain perception.[10,11]

These findings have significant implications for the dental professional. They suggest that tense, fearful patients who flinch and wince at even minor procedures are not just "sissies." Rather, in their highly aroused state these patients actually experience the procedures as more painful than do patients who are less fearful. In one laboratory study, for example, dentally fearful subjects recalled that the pain experienced during experimental tooth shock was more intense than what the non-fearful subjects recalled.[12] It is easy to understand how a vicious cycle can be set in motion. The memory of pain during dental treatment leads to increased anxiety prior to and during subsequent visits. This, in turn, leads to heightened sensitivity to pain, and so on in an upward spiral of fear and pain.

Situational factors that contribute to increased anxiety and sensitivity to pain include the following:

Predictability: Predictable aversive events are less stressful than unpredictable aversive events. Studies have shown that people prefer to be given information about what will happen, even when that knowledge cannot alter the event.[13,14]

Control: Control and predictability are closely associated. In fact, some investigators have suggested that predictability reduces stress by increasing a person's sense of control over an aversive situation. When laboratory subjects are given control over the timing of shocks they will receive, they tolerate higher levels of shock before rating the sensations as uncomfortable. Subsequent loss of control results in lower levels of shock being rated as uncomfortable.[15] For some individuals, perceived lack of control in the operatory is a significant factor in dental fear. One investigator found this to be among the most important factors in maintaining fear among a group of highly fearful, avoidant patients.[16] The widely endorsed practice of telling patients to signal by raising a hand if they need a "rest" indicates that dental professionals recognize the importance of control in relation to pain and anxiety.

Attention: When one is involved in a very absorbing or exciting situation, uncomfortable or even painful stimulation might pass unnoticed. Conversely, the pain from an injury or illness often seems worse at night than it does during the day, when there are activities and events distracting attention from the pain. These examples illustrate the important role of attentional factors in pain perception. In general, directing attention toward painful stimulation causes pain to be perceived as more intense, while directing attention away from painful or uncomfortable sensations helps to reduce perceived discomfort.[17,18]

Manipulation and control of these factors is essential for holding stress and discomfort to a minimum during dental treatment. A variety of methods for controlling these variables are discussed in the section on treating dental fear.

THE ORIGINS OF DENTAL FEAR

To the dental professional, knowledgeable about the benefits of preventive care and enthusiastic about providing such care, statistics concerning fearful, avoidant patients can be baffling. "Why," professionals often ask, "do so many people fear dental treatment?"

Some have suggested that the answer to this question lies within the personality structure, or psyche, of the fearful patient. Surprisingly, only a few studies have explored this issue. From the results of these studies, we can tentatively conclude that fearful patients do not differ from nonfearful patients in terms of dependency, oral activity, or difficulty with authority figures.[19]

Among extremely fearful patients—those who cannot bring themselves to seek dental treatment except in extreme emergencies, and who, even then, refuse treatment unless they are given general anesthesia—there is a higher-than-average incidence of other specific phobias, in addition to dental phobia. Among fearful patients, in comparison with nonfearful patients, we also find a higher number of individuals who are generally tense, anxious, and prone to worry excessively.[20]

In many cases, these tendencies can be traced back to the patient's childhood. In one large study in which dentally phobic children were compared with nonfearful control children, 65 percent of the phobic children were described by their parents as having another disturbance. The most commonly mentioned were "generally worries," "generally highly-strung," and "generally nervous." In marked contrast, only 5 percent of the control children were reported to have another disturbance.[21]

Note that this is by no means the case with *all* severely phobic patients; many such patients—adults and children—appear to be quite well-adjusted, apart from their intense fear of dental treatment. Nor does this mean that all very anxious people are bound to develop dental phobia. However, the findings should certainly alert us to proceed with great care and sensitivity when dealing with patients who seem generally high-strung and tense, especially if they are known to have many fears and worries. By virtue of their personal style, these patients may be predisposed to developing severe dental fear, especially if they undergo what they perceive as a traumatic dental experience.

Traumatic Early Experience

Traumatic dental treatment during childhood or adolescence has, in fact, been implicated as a major source of dental fear in adults.[6,19,20] When fearful adults are asked to recall specific dental events that they consider instrumental in the development of their fear of dentistry, many cite painful dental treatment. An even greater number, however, describe negative aspects of the dental staff's behavior and personal characteristics as significant factors in the development of their dental fear. In one study, for example, half of a group of highly fearful patients made comments such as the following about their former dentists:[22]

> When I was young, my dentist yelled at me to open my mouth, then to close it. In general, he was quite an unlikeable person who did not have a good chairside manner.

> As a child, I went to a dentist who was impersonal, nasty, and was only there to fill my tooth. He didn't seem to give a damn if he hurt me in the process.

Dental assistants fared somewhat better than dentists in this study, but they, too, were the target of some unfavorable comments: 12 percent of the fearful patients specifically mentioned negative aspects of the dental assistant's behavior and personality. This suggests that the assistant does indeed play a role in the development of a patient's attitudes toward dentistry.

These are retrospective reports, and we have no way to evaluate their validity. What is important, however, is the fact that the patients *believed* that they had been poorly or harshly treated, and this belief contributed to their negative attitudes toward dentistry.

The Role of Family and Friends

Another variable on which fearful and nonfearful patients differ is family attitudes toward dentistry. It has been shown that family attitudes toward dentistry play a very significant role in the development of a child's attitudes toward dentistry.[6,19] In a survey in which adolescents and adults were asked to recall important factors in the development of their fear of dentistry, negative expectations learned from family and friends was the most frequently cited recollection.[6]

Stories told by family members who are themselves afraid of the dentist have a powerful effect on a young child's view of dentistry. Even when no frightening tales are told to the child, if a parent or older sibling is fearful, the young child can quickly acquire similar feelings. This is understandable when we consider the critical role of observational learning in the child's development. Anyone who has ever watched a little girl play house or dress up "just like Mommy," or a little boy go through the motions of shaving, "just like Daddy," knows that parents (and, to a lesser extent, older brothers and sisters) are a child's first important models.

Thus, it is not surprising to find that children who are so fearful as to warrant the label "phobic" frequently have parents who themselves feared dental treatment and who have remained very anxious as adult patients. Even among families in which levels of dental anxiety are less pronounced, children of anxious mothers tend to be more anxious and uncooperative at the first dental visit than children whose mothers do not report anxiety concerning the visit.[23]

Peers have also been found to be an important source of children's fear of dentistry.[6] As children grow, they spend less time within the family circle. More time is spent in the company of friends and classmates, who gradually replace the family as the major source of influence on the child's attitudes and opinions. Unfortunately, much of what the child learns about dentistry from other children is negative and frightening in tone. When children are asked to list sources of positive and negative information about dentistry, peers are the most frequently cited source of negative information. In one study, for example, two-thirds of a group of children surveyed identified peers as a source of unfavorable information about the dentist.[24] In contrast, fewer than one-fourth reported learning negative information about the dentist from parents, teachers, nurses, books, or television.

Of what practical use is such information to those interested in the treatment and prevention of dental fear? Findings that underscore the important role of family and friends in the development of dental fear point to the potential utility of programs that use parents, siblings, and peers to teach positive attitudes toward dentistry. Dental professionals, for instance, might devote extra effort to teaching parents how to prepare their children for the first dental visit. Fearless child patients might be used as "models" from whom inexperienced or fearful children can learn to accept treatment with less apprehensiveness. Other examples of programs that involve friends and family in this manner are discussed in Chapter 9.

ASSESSING DENTAL FEAR

It is certainly true that all patients, regardless of their level of dental fear, are entitled to the most considerate and gentle care we can possibly provide; but patients who are highly anxious require special methods if their anxiety is to be reduced to manageable levels. Of course, before special efforts are undertaken to reduce high levels of anxiety, the patient must first be determined to be in need of such efforts. It is necessary, therefore, to have some means of identifying anxious patients and some way in which to assess their level of fear.

Researchers also need methods for accurately measuring dental fear, for without such measures the effectiveness of fear-reduction programs cannot be evaluated. A treatment program cannot be said to be effective unless it can be shown that patients who undergo the program exhibit significant reductions in anxiety following the treatment. Thus, researchers must first be able to measure fear with some degree of confidence in their measures.

On the surface, this would seem to be a simple task. Fear, however, is not something concrete that can be measured with a scale or a yardstick. Fear is a subjective state or experience. It includes:

Thoughts, such as "I'm scared," and "This is awful."

Physiological activation in the autonomic nervous system, including increased perspiration and heart rate.

Overt behavior, such as crying, screaming, trembling, or running away.

For research purposes, responses are often assessed simultaneously in all three channels—thoughts, physiological activity, and overt behavior. To assess fearful thoughts, questionnaires and self-report scales are used. Electrodes placed on the patient's fingers and chest record changes in galvanic skin resistance (GSR), galvanic skin conductance (GSC), and cardiac rate. Sweat gland activity in the hand (palmar sweat index, or PSI) can be monitored by applying a graphite solution which, when dry, can be peeled off, permitting a microscopic examination and count of open sweat pores. Measures of overt behavior include length of time since last dental visit (dental avoidance) and number of broken or cancelled appointments. With child patients, frequency of crying and amount of movement in the dental chair are often used as overt behavioral measures.

For routine use in the dental office, physiological measures are obviously impractical. What self-report measures or observations of patient behavior can be most helpful in the identification of fearful patients?

Dental Fear Questionnaires

Questionnaires are simple to administer, require little time, and can yield valuable information in exchange for very little cost and effort. Two such questionnaires which are often used in research on den-

1. If you had to go to the dentist tomorrow, how would you feel about it?
   a. I would look forward to it as a reasonably enjoyable experience.
   b. I wouldn't care one way or the other.
   c. I would be a little uneasy about it.
   d. I would be afraid that it would be unpleasant and painful.
   e. I would be very frightened of what the dentist might do.
2. When you are waiting in the dentist's office for your turn in the chair, how do you feel?
   a. Relaxed.
   b. A little uneasy.
   c. Tense.
   d. Anxious.
   e. So anxious that I sometimes break out in a sweat or almost feel physically sick.
3. When you are in the dentist's chair waiting while he gets his drill ready to begin working on your teeth, how do you feel?
   a. Relaxed.
   b. A little uneasy.
   c. Tense.
   d. Anxious.
   e. So anxious that I sometimes break out in a sweat or almost feel physically sick.
4. You are in the dentist's chair to have your teeth cleaned. While you are waiting and the dentist is getting out the instruments which he will use to scrape your teeth around the gums, how do you feel?
   a. Relaxed.
   b. A little uneasy.
   c. Tense.
   d. Anxious.
   e. So anxious that I sometimes break out in a sweat or almost feel physically sick.

FIGURE 5-1   Dental Anxiety Scale. From N.L. Corah, Development of a dental anxiety scale, *Journal of Dental Research* 48:596, 1969. Reprinted by permission.

tal fear are also suitable for clinical use. Both have been shown to be valid and reliable measures of dental fear.*

The Dental Anxiety Scale (see Figure 5-1) consists of four items, each with five choices. Responses are scored a = 1 point, b = 2 points, and so on. A score of 13 or 14 on this scale usually indicates that the patient is anxious. Patients who obtain scores of 15 or greater are almost always very anxious.[25]

The Dental Fear Survey, reproduced in Figure 5-2, is another questionnaire which is commonly used to assess dental fear. This questionnaire is somewhat longer than the Dental Anxiety Scale, but it provides

*Validity refers to the extent to which an instrument measures what it is intended to measure; reliability concerns the consistency of an individual's scores across repeated assessment periods with the same instrument. For an excellent discussion of reliability and validity in the context of oral health research, see M.L. Darby and D.M. Bowen, *Research Methods for Oral Health Professionals: An Introduction* (St. Louis: C.V. Mosby, 1980).

Please rate your feeling or reaction on these items using the following scale:

1	2	3	4	5
Never	Once or twice	A few times	Often	Nearly every time

_____ 1. Has fear of dental work ever caused you to put off making an appointment?

_____ 2. Has fear of dental work ever caused you to cancel or not appear for an appointment?

When having dental work done: (Use the following scale)

1	2	3	4	5
Not at all	A little	Somewhat	Much	Very much

_____ 3. My muscles become tense.

_____ 4. My breathing rate increases.

_____ 5. I perspire.

_____ 6. I feel nauseated and sick to my stomach.

_____ 7. My heart beats faster.

Using the scale above, please rate how much fear, anxiety, or unpleasantness each of the following causes you.

_____ 8. Making an appointment for dentistry

_____ 9. Approaching the dentist's office

_____ 10. Sitting in the waiting room

_____ 11. Being seated in the dental operatory

_____ 12. The smell of the dentist's office

_____ 13. Seeing the dentist walk in

_____ 14. Seeing the anesthetic needle

_____ 15. Feeling the needle injected

_____ 16. Seeing the drill

_____ 17. Hearing the drill

_____ 18. Feeling the vibrations of the drill

_____ 19. Having your teeth cleaned

_____ 20. All things considered, how fearful are you of having dental work done?

FIGURE 5-2 Dental Fear Survey. From R.A. Kleinknecht, R.K. Klepac, and L.D. Alexander, Origins and characteristics of fear of dentistry, *Journal of the American Dental Association* 86:842, 1973. Reprinted by permission.

information about specific areas that are especially anxiety-producing for each patient. The patient's score on Item 20 of the Dental Fear Survey is considered to be the total score for the questionnaire. A score of 1 or 2 indicates a lower level of dental fear; a score of 4 or 5 usually indicates that the patient is moderately to highly fearful.[6]

Observation of Patient Behavior

Students sometimes ask, "Why bother with questionnaires? Can't I tell whether a patient is anxious just by observation?" Movies, television, and cartoons depicting the fearful patient cowering in the dental chair or hiding behind the furniture in the reception room support the belief that fearful patients can be identified at a glance. The stereotype of the fearful patient is an individual who paces in the reception room, enters the operatory reluctantly, and fidgets and squirms in the chair. Other behaviors associated with this stereotype include white knuckles from a death grip on the arms of the chair, gasps and groans, and pleas for mercy.

How accurate is this stereotype of the fearful patient? Certainly, some fearful patients do not hesitate to display their anxiety openly, and every dental professional has seen patients who engage in one or more of these behaviors. For the most part, however, fearful patients do *not* move around more or talk more in the dental operatory than nonfearful patients do. In a series of studies, psychologists Kleinknecht and Bernstein used video recording equipment to record the reception room and operatory behavior of high-fear and low-fear patients.[6,26] When trained observers viewed the tapes and coded patient behavior, no differences were found between high-fear and low-fear patients in their behavior in the operatory. Some differences between the groups in reception room behavior were detected, but the differences were not dramatic, and the behavior of fearful patients was far removed from that depicted by cartoonists and comedians.

The most likely explanation for these findings concerning overt behavior of anxious patients is that the behavior of most adults is typically under the strong control of social cues. In many situations, the way in which a person behaves might bear little relation to his feelings about the situation. Who has not had the experience of receiving a gift he considered useless, unattractive, or otherwise disappointing? In such cases, the recipient typically hides his disappointment and assures the giver, "It's just what I wanted." Just as it is considered inappropriate for the recipient to reveal his true feelings in this situation, so most adults are aware that it is inappropriate to thrash about and scream during dental treatment. This awareness of appropriate social behavior serves to inhibit the direct expression of feelings in many such situations.

From this discussion, it should be clear that dental professionals cannot always detect dental fear simply by observing the patient. This, then, is a strong argument in favor of routine use of questionnaires or self-report scales as a means of reliably identifying patients whose fear of dentistry is likely to present problems for themselves and for the dental staff.

REFERENCES

1. Richardson, J.T. Fear: A psychological and a dental problem. *South Carolina Dental Journal* 30:4, 1972.

2. Jenny, J., Frazier, P.J., Bagramian, R.A., and Proshek, J.M. Parents' satisfac-

tion and dissatisfaction with their children's dentist. *Journal of Public Health* 33:211, 1973.

3. Stricker, G., and Howitt, J.W. Physiological recording during simulated dental appointments. *New York State Dental Journal* 31:204, 1965.

4. American Dental Association, Bureau of Economic and Behavioral Research. Dental habits and opinions of the public: Results of a 1978 survey. Chicago, 1979.

5. Ingersoll, B.D., Ingersoll, T.G., McCutcheon, W.R., and Seime, R.J. Behavioral dimensions of dental practice: A national survey. Unpublished manuscript, West Virginia University School of Dentistry, 1979.

6. Kleinknecht, R.A. Dental fear assessment. In *Behavioral dentistry: Proceedings of the First National Conference*, edited by B. Ingersoll, R. Seime, and W. McCutcheon. Morgantown, W.Va.: West Virginia University, 1977.

7. Filewich, R.J., Jackson, E., and Shore, H. Effects of dental fear on efficiency of routine dental procedures. Paper presented at the meeting of the International Association for Dental Research, Chicago, Ill., 1981.

8. Melzack, R., and Dennis, S.G. Neurophysiological foundations of pain. In *The psychology of pain*, edited by R.A. Sternbach. New York: Raven Press, 1971.

9. Sternbach, R.A. Clinical aspects of pain. In *The psychology of pain*, edited by R.A. Sternbach. New York: Raven Press, 1971.

10. Hill, H.E., Kornetsky, C.H., Flanary, H.G., and Wikler, A. Studies on anxiety associated with anticipation of pain: I. Effects of morphine. *Archives of Neurology and Psychiatry* 67:612, 1952.

11. Egbert, L.D., Battit, G.E., Welch, C.E., and Bartlett, M.K. Reduction of postoperative pain by encouragement and instruction of patients. *New England Journal of Medicine* 270:825, 1964.

12. Klepac, R.K., McDonald, M., Hauge, G., and Dowling, J. Reactions to pain among subjects high and low in dental fear. *Journal of Behavioral Medicine* 3:373, 1980.

13. Badia, P., McBane, B., Suter, S., and Lewis, P. Preference behavior in an immediate versus variably delayed shock situation with and without a warning signal. *Journal of Experimental Psychology* 72:847, 1966.

14. Lanzetta, J.T., and Driscoll, J. Preference for information about an uncertain but unavoidable outcome. *Journal of Personality and Social Psychology* 18:157, 1971.

15. Staub, E., Tursky, B., and Schwartz, G.E. Self-control and predictability: Their effects on reactions to aversive stimulation. *Journal of Personality and Social Psychology* 18:157, 1971.

16. Gatchel, R.J. Effectiveness of two procedures for reducing dental fear: Group-administered desensitization and group education and discussion. *Journal of the American Dental Association* 101:634, 1980.

17. Kanfer, F.H., and Goldfoot, D.A. Self-control and tolerance of noxious stimulation. *Psychological Reports* 18:79, 1966.

18. Barber, T.X., and Cooper, B.J. Effects on pain of experimentally induced and spontaneous distraction. *Psychological Reports* 24:647, 1972.

19. Shoben, E.J., and Borland, L. An empirical study of the etiology of dental fears. *Journal of Clinical Psychology* 10:171, 1954.

20. Lautch, H. Dental phobia. *British Journal of Psychiatry* 119:151, 1971.

21. Sermet, O. Emotional and medical factors in child dental anxiety. *Journal of Child Psychology and Psychiatry* 15:313, 1974.

22. Kleinknecht, R.A. Fear of dentistry: Its development, measurement, and implication. In *Advances in behavioral research in dentistry*, edited by P. Weinstein. Seattle, Washington: University of Washington School of Dentistry, 1978.

23. Bailey, P.M., Talbot, A., and Taylor, P.P. A comparison of maternal anxiety levels with anxiety levels manifested in the child dental patient. *Journal of Dentistry for Children* 40:4, 1973.

24. Morgan, P.H., Wright, L.E., Ingersoll, B.D., and Seime, R.J. Children's perceptions of the dental experience. *Journal of Dentistry for Children* 47:242, 1980.

25. Corah, N.L., Gale, E.N., and Illig, S.J. Assessment of a dental anxiety scale. *Journal of the American Dental Association* 97:817, 1978.

26. Kleinknecht, R.A., and Bernstein, D.A. Assessment of dental fear. *Behavior Therapy* 9:626, 1978.

6

Reducing Fear, Pain, and Stress

Even a casual inspection of the dental literature reveals a multitude of articles on the management of dental fear, pain, and stress. If you are a careful reader, you have probably been struck by the fact that a bewildering array of treatment methods are each described by their advocates as the most effective means of minimizing anxiety and discomfort.

Most of these articles, however, are *not* based on controlled scientific investigations. Instead, they are anecdotal reports and subjective impressions based on personal experience. While such reports are certainly thought-provoking and can often provide useful clinical leads, they cannot be used to evaluate the relative merits of one treatment compared to others. Another problem is that we cannot predict from reports such as these which types of patients are most likely to benefit or the success rates we can expect if we use a particular method.

To answer these questions, we must turn to the results of controlled research. Investigations conducted in many dental schools and psychology laboratories across the country have provided promising leads for effective and efficient treatment of dental pain and fear, as we shall discuss in the following sections.

PHARMACOLOGICAL METHODS FOR REDUCING FEAR, PAIN, AND STRESS

There is currently a wide variety of drugs available for the management of acute pain and anxiety. Oral premedication is reasonably safe and simple to administer. The administration of drugs such as Valium (diazepam) and Dalmane (flurazepam hydrochloride), and the use of inhalation sedation with nitrous oxide have helped many tense patients feel more relaxed and comfortable during dental treatment.

Such drugs are a valuable adjunct in the dental armamentarium, but they are not a foolproof solution to all problems, nor are they appropriate for all patients. Some patients cannot take drugs because of allergies, existing medical conditions, or the danger of interaction with other medications. Other patients, aware of reports concerning dangerous long-range effects of some drugs, are reluctant to take medication unless they are seriously ill.

Drugs can be helpful for mildly anxious patients, but they are sometimes of less value with patients who are highly fearful. Dosage can be a problem; the greater the patient's anxiety and fear, the larger the required medication dosage.[1] Small doses, then, may not be sufficient to reduce anxiety, but larger doses increase the chance that the patient will experience unpleasant and even dangerous side effects.

Paradoxical effects of anti-anxiety medication have also been observed with some highly anxious patients. According to Dr. Samuel Dworkin, a researcher trained in both dentistry and psychology:

> . . . Patients highly anxious about general things like loss of control, fear of the unknown, and loss of support view Valium, Demerol, and IVs equally as threatening as operatory procedures. And so, it very often turns out that the very pharmaceutical methods you use for pain control and sedation are not effective in the people who seem to need them the most.[2]

The use of drugs with fearful patients has also been criticized on the grounds that drugs simply make the patient comfortable for the moment. Because the medication does not help him learn to cope with his fears, he never overcomes them. The term *state-dependent learning* is used by psychologists to describe learning that takes place while the individual is in an altered state, such as that induced by drugs or alcohol. Learning that takes place under these conditions does not readily carry over to the undrugged state. For this reason, some have argued that a patient who requires medication to relax during treatment will continue to require medication at subsequent visits. Little is actually known with certainty about this argument as it applies to the fearful dental patient. Controlled longitudinal studies on this subject are needed to resolve the issue.

In summary, while drugs can be quite useful, especially for managing anxiety during emergency situations, many problems accompany their use. Certainly, drugs are not a substitute for nonpharmacological methods of anxiety control.

PREPARATORY MESSAGES: INFORMATION AND EXPOSURE

Dental professionals have long been aware that providing a patient with information about what to expect during treatment can help reduce anxiety and, hence, discomfort. As previously mentioned, predictable aversive events are less stressful than unpredictable aversive events, and anticipatory anxiety about medical and dental procedures can be reduced substantially by providing patients with accurate information about what to expect. In one study, for example, surgical patients who were given preparatory instructions, explanation, and support required far less postoperative pain medication and were ready for discharge earlier than patients who did not receive such preparation.[3]

What are the most important components of an effective preparatory message? Research has shown that patients derive greater benefit from preparatory messages that are *specific* rather than vague, and that emphasize descriptions of *sensations* to be expected rather than procedures to be undertaken.[4,5] For example, one group of investigators prepared children for removal of orthopedic casts, a situation not unlike dental treatment in terms of its use of strange and frightening instruments and procedures. Preparation included exposure to an audio tape of sounds of a saw and descriptions of heat and other sensations accompanying cast removal. During cast removal, these children displayed less fearful, uncooperative behavior than did the children who received only an explanation of the procedures.[6] As we discussed in Chapter 3, you should avoid such threatening words as *pain* and *hurt*, but you can provide accurate descriptions by substituting words like *discomfort, pinch,* and *sting.*

There is also reason to believe that brief explanations might not be as effective in reducing anxiety as preparatory messages that are somewhat *lengthy* and *repetitious.*[7,8] In fact, there are some indications that people who characteristically deal with stress by not thinking about a threatening event actually evidence increased anxiety following a brief preparatory message. When preparatory explanations and instructions are longer and repetitious, however, anxiety is diminished. It is as though longer, repetitious messages provide the patient with an opportunity to "work through" the fear and overcome it. Similarly, longer messages and/or repeated exposure to a single message have been found to be of greater benefit (than short messages or single exposures) to people who characteristically prepare for stressful events by seeking information about, and thinking about, the impending event.

Finally, there is some evidence to indicate that preparatory messages that include *suggestions for coping* with the impending experience can be more helpful than messages that provide only information about the experience. In a study of patients who were about to undergo major surgery, a coping strategy consisting of calming *self*-statements (such as "I'm going to be just fine") and distraction was more effective than simple preparatory explanations in reducing pre- and postoperative stress.[9] Suggestions for helping patients use coping skills are provided later in this chapter.

In light of the findings on effective preparatory messages, films or video tapes would seem to offer an ideal means of providing patients with pretreatment information and exposure to many aspects of the dental experience. Films can convey a great deal of explicit information, including descriptions of the sensations that the patient can expect to experience. In addition, an anxious patient can view a preparatory film or tape several times, if necessary, until the film is no longer upsetting to him. Films can also include suggestions for coping with stressful aspects of the treatment. Finally, films can offer the inexperienced or anxious patient the opportunity to observe other patients successfully coping with dental treatment—a useful strategy known as *modeling.*

Films have many obvious advantages, but a word of caution is in order concerning their use and misuse. Patients should not be left to view preparatory films alone; this is cold, impersonal, and conveys lack of real concern for the patient's welfare. While you need not remain with the patient through the entire film or films, you should check on him frequently and make yourself available to answer any questions.

The value of providing patients with information about, and exposure to, the feared situation has led to the development of two widely used formal treatment methods for reducing fear, both of which incorporate preparatory strategies. These methods, *modeling* and *systematic desensitization,* are discussed in detail in the following sections.

Systematic Desensitization

Systematic desensitization is almost certainly the most widely employed and intensively researched treatment method for reducing irrational fears and phobias. Use of the method was first reported in the psychological literature in 1924, when Mary Cover Jones desensitized a young child to fear of rabbits by feeding the child ice cream while gradually moving a live rabbit closer and closer to him.

Jones' approach was later expanded and refined by Dr. Joseph Wolpe. Dr. Wolpe's work—first with experimental animals made fearful by electric shock; later with fearful humans—is largely responsible for the set of procedures that are now known as systematic desensitization.

In developing his fear-reduction procedures, Dr. Wolpe reasoned that, "If a response inhibiting anxiety can be made to occur in the presence of anxiety-evoking stimuli, it will weaken the bond between these stimuli and the anxiety."[10] Because relaxation is obviously a response that is antagonistic to anxiety (a person cannot feel relaxed and anxious at the same time), Wolpe focused on relaxation as an anxiety-inhibiting response. Fearful patients were trained in *progressive relaxation*, a simple and efficient method of producing comfortable levels of relaxation.

Wolpe discovered that actual contact with the feared object was not necessary for fear reduction to occur; it was sufficient to have patients visualize themselves in fear-evoking situations. In order to help patients remain relaxed in the presence of the fear-evoking object or situation, Wolpe introduced the fear stimuli gradually. For each patient, fear-producing situations were rank-ordered from the least frightening to the most frightening. For example, a snake-phobic person might describe "Looking at pictures of snakes in a book" as a low-fear event, while "Holding a live snake" would certainly rank as one of the most frightening situations for him.

While in a relaxed state, patients were instructed to visualize scenes from their lists, beginning with the lowest (least frightening) item. Patients gradually progressed to more frightening items and were finally able to remain relaxed while visualizing even the most frightening items on their lists. Generalization to the real situation occurred, so that patients no longer responded with excessive fear when actually placed in situations that previously had been very frightening to them.

During the 1970s, a virtual flood of research on systematic desensitization poured from university laboratories and clinics. Investigators applied the approach to a broad range of irrational fears, including fear of snakes, insects, animals, heights, water, darkness, public speaking, members of the opposite sex, flying, loud noises, and injections. The patient populations studied ranged from college sophomores who had fears of snakes or spiders to psychiatric patients who were severely disabled by their irrational fears. Success rates reported were consistently high, and the method itself was found to be simple to employ and far less time-consuming than traditional forms of psychotherapy for phobias.

Researchers seeking ways to manage dental fear were quick to seize upon systematic desensitization as a potentially useful treatment for fearful patients. The first reported application of systematic desensitization to dental fear appeared in 1969.[11] The patient was a 32-year-old man with a history of dental fear so intense that it prevented him from seeking dental treatment for many years, despite repeated painful toothaches. After nine one-hour sessions of systematic desensitization, the patient made and kept dental appointments, completed all necessary dental treatment (including restorations and extractions), and even described dental treatment as "relaxing."

The results of other case reports and controlled studies have also supported the usefulness of systematic desensitization as a treatment for reducing dental fear with some fearful patients. Investigators report success rates (defined as the number of patients who obtain nonemergency dental treatment following participation in a program of systematic desensitization) in the range of about one-half to two-thirds* of severely phobic patients.[12,13]

Extensive training in psychology is not required in order to employ systematic desensitization successfully with fearful dental patients. Traditional desensitization procedures are time-consuming to administer, however, and it is unlikely that they could be employed routinely in a busy dental office.

A more practical alternative to traditional procedures is to permit fearful patients to view videotaped scenes, arranged in graduated order from least fear-producing to most fear-producing. (See Appendix A for a sample list of dental fear scenes.) When this method was used with a group of intensely fearful dental avoiders, two-thirds subsequently made and kept dental appointments.[12] The method is easier and less expensive to implement than it might appear to be at first glance. Reliable, easy-to-operate video recording equipment for home use is widely available at reasonable cost. The purchase of such equipment for a dental practice is a tax-deductible business expense, and the equipment can be used for a variety of purposes, as we will discuss in later sections.

A less costly approach is to provide the patient with an audio tape cassette of relaxation instructions and scenes from a standard list of dental fear scenes. (See Appendixes A and B.) At the initial examination visit or at the prophylaxis visit, the patient could be given the tape and instructions for its use. In the interval before the first restorative visit, the patient could listen to the tape several times in his own home.

Modeling

Just as people can learn maladaptive behavior patterns by observing others, research has shown that they can learn more adaptive attitudes and behavior through the same observational processes. The use of fearless individuals as "models" to help fearful individuals overcome their fears has been found to be effective with a wide variety of fears in children and adults.[14] In both clinical and laboratory studies, filmed modeling has proved as effective as the use of live models—an important point, as live models are not always readily available in the opera-

---

*As these figures represent successful treatment of extremely fearful, long-term dental avoiders, we should expect higher rates of improvement among patients who, although quite fearful, can at least make and keep a dental appointment.

tory. In the dental setting, modeling has been studied extensively as a means of helping inexperienced children prepare for dental treatment. Researchers have studied the effectiveness of modeling in reducing dental fear with adult dental patients.[12] In the study, highly fearful dental avoiders were treated either with filmed modeling or with participant modeling, a procedure which involved observing a live model, followed by immediate practice of each step after it was modeled. After treatment, over half of the patients in the filmed modeling group and almost two-thirds of those in the participant modeling group spontaneously sought dental treatment.

These figures are encouraging, but perhaps the most interesting findings from this study concern the performance of patients in the so-called attention-placebo control group, which was included as a means of controlling for, or ruling out, nonspecific factors associated with participation in *any* fear reduction program. Patients in this group were told that the treatment would help them learn to remain calm and relaxed during dental treatment, but the procedures actually had no presumed active therapeutic ingredients. Nevertheless, after completing the bogus treatment, two-thirds of the patients in this group made and kept dental appointments!

What do these findings mean? The authors suggest that one's belief that one can cope with a stressful situation—a belief fostered by all of the treatment methods used in this study, including the bogus treatment—is a critical factor in reducing fear and avoidance of that particular situation.

Combined procedures. The findings we have just discussed lead us to speculate that procedures that combine a modeling component (to provide explicit information about the dental experience) together with a coping strategy that the patient can use (such as the relaxation component of systematic desensitization) might be more effective than either component used alone. In fact, research evidence supports this notion. In two controlled studies, fearful, avoidant patients were taught relaxation procedures and were then shown modeling films while relaxed. In both studies, success rates of 78 percent were obtained—higher than when either strategy was used alone.[15,16]

In a more recent study, one group of dental avoiders received traditional systematic desensitization (relaxation paired with visualization of graduated fear scenes) followed by specific instructions in a variety of methods for coping with stress during dental treatment.[17] The methods included the following:

Patients were instructed to use relaxation to cope with dental treatment.

Open discussion of specific fears with the dentist was encouraged. To provide patients with a feeling of control, they were instructed to signal the dentist to stop if they felt the need for a brief pause.

A second group of patients participated in an educational program in which information about dental procedures was combined with suggestions for coping. Both groups showed improvement; after treatment, 88 percent of the patients in the desensitization-plus-coping group and 100 percent of those in the educational group had obtained dental care.

In summary, we can conclude that an information-exposure approach is useful for reducing dental fear and avoidance for some patients. For these patients, exposure appears to provide an opportunity to plan or rehearse coping strategies already in their repertoires. Other patients, however, seem to require assistance in developing and using coping skills. For these patients, specific instructions for coping with stress during dental treatment appear to be necessary in order for maximum benefits to accrue. Methods for helping patients cope with dental stress are discussed in the following section.

COPING STRATEGIES

The coping strategies to be discussed in this section include relaxation, biofeedback, and distraction. Because patients are individuals, it is likely that no single coping strategy or technique will be of benefit to everyone. While many patients can benefit from relaxation procedures, for example, others equate relaxation with loss of control and actually experience increased distress as they begin to relax tense muscles. For such patients, a distraction strategy would probably prove more beneficial.

Relaxation

Progressive relaxation, the method used for teaching muscle relaxation in systematic desensitization programs, is a verbal technique originally developed in 1938 and later modified by Wolpe.[18] In the laboratory, muscular relaxation produced with this method has been found to be helpful in lowering anxiety during stressful situations, especially with highly anxious people.[19] It has also been shown to result in increased tolerance for experimentally induced pain[20] and to be of benefit to some individuals with myofascial-pain-dysfunction syndrome.[21]

In a preceding section, we suggested that the relaxation component of systematic desensitization might be effective not only as a means of decreasing anticipatory anxiety, but also as a coping skill that could be used during actual dental treatment. In fact, there is considerable evidence to support this notion. When fearful dental patients are given a series of relaxation training sessions prior to restorative treatment, the result is muscle tension and anxiety decrease significantly during subsequent restorative visits.[22]

These results are promising, but a practical problem is immediately obvious: Between-visit training sessions involve costly demands on office space and professional time. Thus, audiotaped instructions for progressive relaxation might be a more practical alternative to "live" training sessions. Patients can use these tapes to learn and practice progressive relaxation at home. Such tapes are available commercially, or, as we have suggested, you can easily make your own (see Appendix A).

Another inexpensive alternative is simply to have the patient listen, through headphones, to a relaxation tape during actual dental treatment. This approach yields very good results: Patients who listen to a relaxation tape during restorative treatment show significant reductions in anxiety and self-reported discomfort.[23] The effects of listening to such a tape appear to be especially beneficial to highly anxious patients.

Biofeedback

Increases in physiological arousal are one component of anxiety. The physiological change reported as most common and most intense by patients undergoing dental treatment is increased muscle tension.[24] Other frequently noted changes include increases in salivation, heart rate, perspiration, and respiration.

Responses such as increased heart rate, salivation, perspiration, and other physiological changes under the control of the autonomic nervous system were, for many years, believed to be beyond the range of voluntary control. During the 1960s, however, scientists exploring self-control of physiological responses found that many so-called involuntary responses could be brought under voluntary control by means of biofeedback procedures.

Biofeedback has been defined as "the use of electronic monitoring instruments to record and display physiological processes within the body . . . to make this otherwise unavailable information available to the individual."[25] Using this information, often presented in the form of a signal light or tone, patients can be trained to alter their level of physiological activity.

Biofeedback has been used in the treatment of a variety of medical disorders, including headache, hypertension, Raynaud's disease, and insomnia. In the dental context, a variety of biofeedback procedures have been used to reduce patient tension and discomfort during dental treatment. Several investigators have studied the use of electromyographic (EMG) biofeedback to reduce muscle tension—a logical target, in light of the prevalence of this anxiety-related response among patients undergoing dental treatment.[22,26,27] In one study, biofeedback was combined with progressive relaxation procedures in an attempt to enhance the patient's ability to relax.[26] A successful outcome was reported with ten highly anxious patients who had avoided dental treatment for one to fifteen years. It has also been reported that when EMG biofeedback and progressive relaxation procedures are compared, both procedures are equally effective with dentally anxious patients, and both produce significant reductions in muscle tension and anxiety levels during dental treatment.[22]

This suggests that EMG biofeedback is a useful method for reducing tension and anxiety during dental treatment. However, although the instruments and procedures are fairly simple to use, the amount of time required for training patients in biofeedback, at least as the procedures have been described above, would seem to make this method impractical for routine office use.

Mindful of the time constraints of a busy dental practice, dentist-psychologist Richard Hirschman explored the use of brief EMG training sessions.[27] Using a procedure that required only a single eight-minute training session, Dr. Hirschman trained highly anxious dental patients to decrease muscle tension in the forearm. This training procedure produced decreased anxiety during treatment; in contrast, a group of patients who did not receive biofeedback showed *increased* anxiety. In addition, biofeedback patients experienced the restorative procedures as less stressful than they had anticipated, while patients who did not undergo biofeedback training experienced the procedures as *more* stressful than anticipated.

Dr. Hirschman and his research group have also developed a simple technique known as "paced respiration," a procedure which involves teaching patients to pace their breathing with a signal light or tone.[28] When highly anxious patients are taught to pace their respiration at a slower-than-normal rate (eight cycles of inhalation-exhalation a minute), they evaluate dental treatment as less unpleasant than do patients who breathe at a normal rate (16 cycles a minute) or a faster-than-normal rate (24 cycles a minute). This simple but effective technique is ideal for routine use in any dental office, as it requires only a tape recorder and an easily made tape recording of the word *inhale* repeated at 7.5-second intervals. (Patients are told that they can exhale when they wish.)

Increases in heart rate have been described by many patients who are fearful of dental treatment; Hirschman's group has also studied the use of heart rate feedback to reduce anxiety.[28] During their investigation of this method, some individuals were deliberately given inaccurate feedback; that is, signals indicated decreases in heart rate when increases were actually occurring, or increases when heart rate was decreasing. Interestingly, accuracy of feedback had no effect on outcome. Regardless of the accuracy of the feedback, individuals who received feedback indicating that their heart rate was decreasing rated dental events as less unpleasant than did individuals who were given feedback indicating that their heart rate was increasing. These fascinating results suggest that the actual magnitude or direction of physiological change— or even whether change occurs at all—might not be important, as long as the patient *believes* that the appropriate change is taking place.

Indeed, some behavioral scientists have speculated that biofeedback procedures might prove to be the "ultimate placebo."[29] As one explains:

> Biofeedback may simply be effective because of its ability to focus the patient on his physiological condition and at the same time, focus him away from stress-producing sources of tension. Any technique that teaches the patient to be aware of the debilitating effects of negative thoughts and feelings is likely to possess some therapeutic value.[25]

Of greater practical interest for our purposes is the fact that biofeedback procedures do appear to be of benefit to highly anxious patients undergoing dental treatment. Reliable, compact equipment is available at reasonable cost, and the procedures are simple, brief, and efficient.*

Distraction

Several lines of evidence point to distraction as a useful method for reducing pain, discomfort, and stress. Anecdotally, there have been many reports through the years of people who have managed to control pain by focusing their attention on other matters. For example, the German philosopher Kant, who suffered from painful attacks of gout, is reported to have relieved his pain by concentrating on difficult philosophical problems.[30]

In the laboratory, when subjects are instructed to focus their at-

---

*Additional information about biofeedback procedures and equipment can be obtained from The Biofeedback Society of America, 4301 Owens Street, Wheat Ridge, Colorado 80033. A useful text is *Biofeedback: Principles and Practice for Clinicians*, edited by J.V. Basmajian (Williams and Wilkins, 1979).

tention on distracting material or tasks, pain perception is reduced. In one study, experimental pain was produced by attaching a heavy weight to the subject's finger.[31] Subjects were told to listen carefully to an exciting tape-recorded story and to remember as many details as possible. This distracting task resulted in marked reductions in pain reported by the subjects.

Other distracting material that has proved helpful in reducing pain perception includes slides, movies, and word or number tasks.[32,33] Researchers have also obtained good results by instructing subjects to produce their own "internal distractors"—to, for example, imagine exciting or pleasurable events.[34]

In the dental setting, distraction in the form of "audio-analgesia" has been found to be helpful to many patients. Audio-analgesia involves presenting music and white noise (masking sound) to the patient through earphones. The patient is instructed to increase the volume of the music and/or the noise if he feels any discomfort. Although this interesting technique did not live up to early claims of complete pain suppression in all patients, it has proved useful for reducing stress and discomfort for many patients, especially when accompanied by enthusiastic suggestions concerning its beneficial effects.[35]

A research team headed by Doctors Norman Corah and Elliott Gale has been particularly creative in developing distracting material appropriate for use in the dental operatory.[23,36] Working with a group of highly anxious patients, these investigators obtained excellent results with a video table tennis game mounted near the ceiling, with controls on the arm of the chair. Patients permitted to play "against the house" during restorative treatment found the game enjoyable. They also rated themselves as significantly less anxious and the dental procedures as less uncomfortable.

Corah and Gale's group has also explored the use of videotaped programs and audiotaped material with patients undergoing dental treatment. Viewing videotaped programs produced results comparable to those obtained with the video game. Beneficial effects of listening to an audiotaped comedy program were less marked, although some patients were helped by this easily implemented approach.

In summary, permitting patients to watch television, listen to tapes, or play video games appears to be a simple but excellent method for promoting patient comfort and relaxation during dental treatment. Use of these enjoyable distractors should not be limited to fearful patients. Even patients who experience minimal dental fear become bored during dental treatment, and tapes or games can help relieve boredom during long sessions in the chair.

HYPNOSIS

For well over a century, hypnosis has been a subject of considerable controversy among scientists and members of the health care professions. Although the efficacy of hypnosis in relieving pain (especially pain associated with surgical procedures) was demonstrated repeatedly during the first part of the nineteenth century, strong opposition to hypnosis was widespread. In fact, many physicians who used hypnosis were severely censured by their peers. Some, such as John Elliott, a member of the medical faculty at University College in London, even lost their positions at colleges, universities, and hospitals as a result of practicing hypnosis on their patients.

Resistance to hypnosis can be traced in part to the manner in which it was introduced to European society. During the late eighteenth century, Franz Anton Mesmer, a flamboyant Viennese physician, intrigued Parisians with displays of "magnetism." Patients suffering from various illnesses reportedly experienced dramatic cures, which Mesmer attributed to the beneficial effects of magnetic fluids. Mesmer attracted a great deal of attention and drew many followers, but there were also many who believed him to be a charlatan. A royal commission was appointed by the French king to study magnetism, or mesmerism, as it came to be called. The report of this commission discredited Mesmer and denounced mesmerism as unscientific. As a result, interest in hypnosis waned and finally, with the introduction of chemical anesthetics such as ether and chloroform, all but vanished.

Even today, many people remain skeptical about the value and validity of hypnosis. This skepticism probably has been fostered by movies, television programs and stage show hypnosis, all of which usually depict hypnosis as a mysterious force that a person in a hypnotic trance is unable to resist or disobey. Such myths and misconceptions have certainly impeded the acceptance of hypnosis as a legitimate clinical tool.

The past few decades have, nevertheless, seen a renewed surge of interest in hypnosis within medicine, dentistry, and psychology. Hypnosis is now generally regarded as a legitimate subject for scientific investigation and as a useful adjunct in the clinician's armamentarium. In 1955, the American Medical Association sanctioned the teaching of hypnosis in American medical schools. Hypnosis has also been accepted in dental education. In just seven years, the number of dental schools that include hypnosis in the curriculum doubled, from one-fourth in 1973 to almost half of all American dental schools in 1980.[37]

The dental profession has, in fact, played an important role in the current revival of interest in hypnosis. Dentists pioneered the clinical use of hypnosis and have discovered many applications for it in the practice of dentistry. The following is an example of hypnosis applied to a patient with marked fear of dentistry and inability to tolerate local anesthesia:

> A 36-year-old woman had previously reacted to procaine with edema of the face and body, urticaria, nausea, and vomiting. As a result, even minor dental procedures had been carried out under general anesthesia. Because of her unfortunate experiences, she had refused to return to her dentist; by now most of her teeth had developed cavities. She needed a series of sessions with her dentist, and it was judged impractical to place her under a general anesthetic each time. . . . After a discussion, hypnosis was induced; she proved to be an excellent subject and was soon capable of reaching a profound hypnotic state. Thereafter, on five separate occasions, dental procedures lasting approximately two hours were successfully performed. On all five occasions, the patient achieved analgesia through hypnotic suggestion alone. She was free of all pain and apprehensiveness. Eventually her fears of dentistry were greatly diminished and she could accept minor procedures without hypnosis.[38]

How are effects such as these achieved? How does hypnosis work? As a result of careful study, hypnosis has been revealed not as a mysterious "power" or "force," but rather as a means of focusing the patient's attention and increasing receptivity to therapeutic suggestions. Although researchers disagree on the exact mechanism by which the effects of hypnosis and hypnosis-like procedures are produced, a large body of clinical and experimental evidence attests to beneficial effects. Many studies, for example, have documented significant alterations in blood flow and reduced blood loss during surgery,[39] as well as marked reduction in pain of laboratory, clinical, and surgical origin.[40,41,42]

As we might expect, individuals differ in the ease and rapidity with which they are able to enter hypnotic trances and respond to suggestion. Thus, hypnosis, like all of the techniques and approaches to patient management we have discussed, is not necessarily suitable for all patients, nor is its use appropriate in all situations. Acknowledged experts in the field of hypnosis agree:

> Hypnosis should be considered a tool to be used wisely and with discrimination, only when circumstances are appropriate. It may be used as the sole anesthetic, or, more often, in conjunction with chemical anesthetics or analgesics. Just as the anesthesiologist has a variety of chemical agents to be used with discretion, so too hypnosis has its appropriate and inappropriate uses.[38]

With this caveat in mind, we conclude that clinical and research evidence strongly supports the usefulness of hypnosis for relieving pain, fear, and stress in medical and dental settings. Hypnosis is a noninvasive procedure. There is little risk involved in its use, and the benefits are often gratifying to both professional and patient.

REFERENCES

1. Malamed, S.F. Pharmacology and therapeutics of anxiety and pain control. In *Textbook of pediatric dentistry*, edited by R.L. Braham and M.E. Morris. Baltimore, Md.: Williams and Wilkins, 1980.

2. Dworkin, S.F. Quoted in Weinstein, P., and Getz, T. *Changing human behavior: Strategies for preventive dentistry*. Chicago: SRA, 1978.

3. Egbert, L.D., Battit, G.E., Welch, C.E., and Bartlett, M.K. Reduction of postoperative pain by encouragement and instruction of patients. *New England Journal of Medicine* 270:825, 1964.

4. Johnson, J.E., and Rice, V.H. Sensory and distress components of pain: Implications for the study of clinical pain. *Nursing Research* 23:203, 1974.

5. Johnson, J.E., and Leventhal, H. Effects of accurate expectations and behavioral instructions on reactions during a noxious medical examination. *Journal of Personality and Social Psychology* 29:710, 1974.

6. Johnson, J.E., Kirchoff, K.T., and Endress, M.P. Altering children's distress behavior during orthopedic cast removal. *Nursing Research* 24:404, 1975.

7. Shipley, R.H., Butt, J.H., Horwitz, B., and Farbry, J.E. Preparation for a stressful medical procedure: Effect of amount of stimulus pre-exposure and coping style. *Journal of Consulting and Clinical Psychology* 46:499, 1978.

8. Shipley, R.H., Butt, J.H., and Horwitz, E.A. Preparation to re-experience a stressful medical examination: Effect of repetitive videotape exposure and coping style. *Journal of Consulting and Clinical Psychology* 47:485, 1979.

9. Langer, E.J., Janis, I.L., and Wolfer, J.A. Reduction of psychological stress in surgical patients. *Journal of Experimental and Social Psychology* 11:155, 1975.

10. Wolpe, J. *The practice of behavior therapy*. Elmsford, N.Y.: Pergamon Press, 1973.

11. Gale, E.N., and Ayer, W.A. Treatment of dental phobias. *Journal of the American Dental Association* 78:1304, 1969.

12. Bernstein, D.A., and Kleinknecht, R.A. Comparative evaluation of three social-learning approaches to the reduction of dental fear. In *Clinical research in behavioral dentistry: Proceedings of the Second National Conference on Behavioral Dentistry*, edited by B.D. Ingersoll and W.R. McCutcheon. Morgantown, W.Va.: West Virginia University, 1979.

13. Klepac, R.K. Successful treatment of avoidance of dentistry by desensitization or by increasing pain tolerance. *Journal of Behavior Therapy and Experimental Psychiatry* 6:307, 1975.

14. Bandura, A. *Principles of behavior modification*. New York: Holt, Rinehart & Winston, 1969.

15. Shaw, D.W., and Thoreson, C.E. Effects of modeling and desensitization in reducing dental phobia. *Journal of Counseling Psychology* 20:415, 1974.

16. Wroblewski, P.F., Jacob, T., and Rehm, L.P. The contribution of relaxation to symbolic modeling in the modification of dental fears. *Behavior Research and Therapy* 15:113, 1977.

17. Gatchel, R.J. Effectiveness of two procedures for reducing dental fear: Group-administered desensitization and group education and discussion. *Journal of the American Dental Association* 101:634, 1980.

18. Jacobsen, E. *Progressive relaxation.* Chicago: University of Chicago Press, 1938.

19. Wilson, A., and Wilson, A.S. Psychophysiological and learning correlates of anxiety and induced muscle relaxation. *Psychophysiology* 6:740, 1970.

20. Bobey, M.J., and Davidson, P.O. Psychological factors affecting pain tolerance. *Journal of Psychosomatic Research* 14:371, 1970.

21. Gessel, A.H., and Adlerman, M.M. Management of myofascial pain dysfunction syndrome of the temporomandibular joint by tension control training. *Psychosomatics* 12:302, 1971.

22. Miller, M.P., Murphy, P.J., and Miller, T.P. Comparison of electromyographic feedback and progressive relaxation in treating circumscribed anxiety stress reaction. *Journal of Consulting and Clinical Psychology* 46:1291, 1978.

23. Corah, N.L., Gale, E.N., and Illig, S.J. The use of relaxation and distraction to reduce psychological stress during dental procedures. *Journal of the American Dental Association* 98:390, 1979.

24. Kleinknecht, R.A. Dental fear assessment. In *Behavioral dentistry: Proceedings of the First National Conference,* edited by B. Ingersoll, R. Seime, and W. McCutcheon. Morgantown, W.Va.: West Virginia University, 1977.

25. Bakal, D.A. *Psychology and medicine: Psychobiological dimensions of health and illness.* New York: Springer Publishing Co., 1979.

26. Carlsson, S.G., Linde, A., and Ohman, A. Reduction of tension in fearful dental patients. *Journal of the American Dental Association* 101:638, 1980.

27. Hirschman, R. Physiological feedback and stress reduction. In B.D. Ingersoll (chair), Behavioral approaches to dental fear, pain, and stress. Symposium presented at the meeting of the Society of Behavioral Medicine, New York, November, 1980.

28. Hirschman, R., Young, D., and Nelson, C. Physiologically based techniques for stress reduction. In *Clinical research in behavioral dentistry: Proceedings of the Second National Conference on Behavioral Dentistry,* edited by B.D. Ingersoll and W.R. McCutcheon. Morgantown, W.Va.: West Virginia University, 1979.

29. Stroebel, C.F., and Glueck, B.C. Biofeedback treatment in medicine and psychiatry: An ultimate placebo? In *Biofeedback: Behavioral medicine,* edited by L. Birk. New York: Grune & Stratton, 1973.

30. Ischlondsky, N.E. *Brain and behavior.* St. Louis, Mo.: C.V. Mosby, 1949.

31. Barber, T.X. Effects of hypnotic induction, suggestion of anesthesia and distraction on subjective and physiological responses to pain. Paper presented at the meeting of the Eastern Psychological Association, Philadelphia, 1969.

32. Kanfer, F.H., and Goldfoot, D.A. Self-control and tolerance of noxious stimulation. *Psychological Reports* 18:79, 1966.

33. Barber, T.X., and Cooper, B.J. Effects on pain of experimentally-induced and spontaneous distraction. *Psychological Reports* 24:647, 1972.

34. Chaves, J., and Barber, T. Cognitive strategies, experimenter modeling, and expectation in the attenuation of pain. *Journal of Abnormal Psychology* 83:356, 1974.

35. Melzack, R. *The puzzle of pain.* New York: Basic Books, 1973.

36. Corah, N.L., Gale, E.N., Pace, L.F., and Seyrek, S.K. Comparison of three distraction techniques in reducing dental stress. Paper presented at the meeting of the International Association for Dental Research, Chicago, March, 1981.

37. Simpson, R.B., Dedmon, H., Logan, N., and Jakobsen, J. Hypnosis in dental education: A survey of U.S. dental schools. Unpublished manuscript, University of Iowa College of Dentistry, 1981.

38. Hilgard, E.R. Hypnosis and pain. In *The psychology of pain*, edited by R.A. Sternbach, New York: Raven Press, 1978.

39. Chaves, J.F., Whilden, D., and Roller, N. Hypnosis in dental behavioral science: Control of surgical and post-surgical bleeding. In *Clinical research in behavioral dentistry: Proceedings of the Second National Conference on Behavioral Dentistry*, edited by B.D. Ingersoll and W.R. McCutcheon. Morgantown, W.Va.: West Virginia University, 1979.

40. Barber, T.X., and Hahn, K.W. Physiological and subjective responses to pain-producing stimulation under hypnotically suggested and waking imagined "analgesia." *Journal of Abnormal and Social Psychology* 65:411, 1962.

41. Melzack, R., and Perry, C. Self-regulation of pain: The use of alpha-feedback and hypnotic training for the control of chronic pain. *Experimental Neurology* 46:452, 1975.

42. Bowers, K.S., and van der Meulen, A. A comparison of psychological and chemical techniques in the control of dental pain. Paper presented at the meeting of the Society for Clinical and Experimental Hypnosis, Boston, 1972.

7

The Problem of Nonadherence

In the not-too-distant past, little scientific information was available concerning the pathogenesis of periodontal disease or dental caries, and the scope of dental care was, for the most part, limited to providing remedial treatment. Since that time, great scientific and technological progress has been made. Periodontal disease and caries are now known to be preventable, and preventive activities have assumed an important role in current dental practice. Despite preventive efforts, however, dental disease remains the most prevalent of all diseases. It is estimated that virtually *all* people (close to 99 percent) exhibit dental caries, and over 80 percent of the adult population suffer from periodontal disease.[1] The average DMF index of adults between the ages of 25 and 34 is 18,[2] and over half of the population 55 years of age and older are edentulous.[3]

These grim statistics are well known to dental professionals, as are statistics concerning preventive activities:

In a given year, only about half of the population visit the dentist; 22 percent report no visits for three years or longer.[4]

Almost one-third (30 percent) of children under the age of 17 have never been to the dentist.[5]

Less than half of the population have ever used dental floss; less than 5 percent report flossing on a daily basis.[6]

Thus, although the technology for controlling dental disease is available, it is clear that a major problem remains: How can we convince people to use this technology—to seek routine care, to control their diets, and to brush and floss regularly?

The dental professional, of course, must face this problem on a daily basis, and few claim to have solved it. In a national survey, three-quarters of the dentists asked reported problems with patients who do not engage in sound home care practices; over two-thirds described patients who appear to know or care very little about the benefits of preventive care.[7] Dentists in practice for less than ten years were especially likely to complain of the latter problem, probably because younger dentists have been exposed to heavy emphasis on prevention in the dental school curriculum and are, therefore, concerned about problems in this area. No published statistics are available, but it seems safe to assume that the situation is much the same for the dental hygienist.

Of course, oral health care professionals are not alone: Patients who do not follow health care recommendations are encountered by all health care professionals. One writer who reviewed the results of several large-scale studies concluded that between 30 and 70 percent of all recommendations for medication, home care, exercise, diet, and the like were *not* followed by patients.[8] Another researcher studying patient cooperation with recommendations for professional preventive care and home care reported that only about one-third of the patients he studied could be considered highly cooperative, while approximately one-fourth were considered completely uncooperative.[9] Thus, of every ten patients you see, only about three will follow your recommendations for home care and professionally provided preventive care. Seven of the ten will disregard some, or all, of your recommendations.

What, if anything, can be done about this frustrating state of affairs? Before turning to a discussion of ways in which adherence to preventive regimens might be improved, let us first examine some of the principal factors associated with patient cooperation and compliance.

FACTORS ASSOCIATED WITH ADHERENCE
TO PREVENTIVE REGIMENS

Why do people fail to do what they know they ought to do? Can we predict who will follow our recommendations and who will disregard them? In a comprehensive review of the enormous literature on this subject, one writer identified more than 200 factors that have been associated with adherence to treatment and preventive regimens.[10] Of this number, only a few have consistently been found to be useful predictors of adherence.

Patient Characteristics

When health care professionals are asked why patients do not adhere to treatment and preventive regimens, two-thirds cite "uncooperative personalities" as the reason.[9] Researchers, too, have speculated that the nonadhering patient has passive-aggressive traits or has trouble with authority figures. Research, however, has not supported these assumptions: In studies comparing adhering patients with nonadhering patients, no personality differences have been found to distinguish between the two.[10]

On the other hand, educational level, income, and occupational status have all been found to be positively associated with preventive dental visits.[11,4] For example, one large-scale survey showed that among patients earning $25,000 or more, almost half reported having seen a dentist within the preceding six months, while only one-fourth of those earning less than $7000 had done so.[4] A similar pattern was observed regarding educational level: Almost half of the college graduates surveyed reported a dental visit within the preceding six months, but this figure dropped to 19 percent among those with less than a high-school degree. This survey also showed that whites had a slight but definite tendency toward more recent dental visits than nonwhites, and working women had more recent visits than homemakers.

Of course, educational level, occupational status, and race are all associated with income, and, indeed, many people who do not obtain routine preventive care cite cost as a major obstacle. Even when costs are covered by third-party payment, however, these differences do not disappear.[12] Further, a similar pattern of differences in home care practices has been found among groups differing in educational level and income. College-educated people, for example, are more than twice as likely to use dental floss than people with less than a high-school education.[4] Therefore, cost alone cannot explain the differences among groups.

Differences in health belief systems have also been found to distinguish between people who engage in preventive oral health activities and those who do not. A large body of research on the so-called Health Belief Model indicates that people who engage in preventive health activities believe that:

They are susceptible to a specific disease.

Contracting the disease would be serious.

They can prevent the disease or make it less serious, if contracted, by engaging in preventive activities.[13,14]

In an early application of this model to dental behavior, factory workers with free dental care for themselves and their families were interviewed.[14] Of those who believed that they were highly susceptible to dental disease, that dental disease is serious, and that they could take preventive action, 80 percent had made preventive dental visits within the preceding three years. Of those who scored low on these beliefs, none had made a preventive visit within the preceding three years.

This study and several others have shown that there is a relationship between health beliefs and preventive behavior. A great many researchers and clinicians have interpreted this relationship to mean that health beliefs *cause* health behavior and have focused their efforts on changing beliefs through educational programs, in the hope that behavior change would follow. The general lack of success of such efforts, which will be discussed in a later section, suggests that the relationship between beliefs and behavior might not be as direct as it appears: Beliefs cannot be used to predict behavior, and changing an individual's beliefs does not necessarily result in changes in behavior.

Provider Characteristics

One variable that has consistently emerged as an important factor in determining adherence is the relationship between patient and health care provider. Studies have repeatedly shown that patients who are satisfied with the care they receive and who perceive the provider as caring are more likely to follow the professional's recommendations and instructions than are patients who are dissatisfied.[15]

The status and perceived expertise of the provider also appear to be related to adherence. For example, patients are more likely to follow the advice of a psychologist when he is referred to as "doctor" than when he is called "mister."[16] This variable was examined in the dental setting in a study comparing patient adherence to advice given by dentists, dental assistants, and secretaries.[17] Two dentists and a dental assistant and secretary employed in each of their offices were each assigned a group of 30 patients and instructed to tell the patients the following: "There is a new dental care booklet I think you should read. It is free of charge if you just fill out this card with your name and address and drop it in a mailbox." The cards were prestamped, addressed, and covertly marked to indicate the identity of the communicator. The return rates for both of the dentists were significantly higher (60 and 47 percent) than the return rates for the dental assistants (43 and 27 percent), who in turn fared better than the secretaries (23 and 13 percent).

As only two members of each group—dentists, dental assistants, and secretaries—comprised the sample used in this study, we must use considerable caution in drawing general conclusions based on the results. Nevertheless, this study suggests that assistants, at least, are at a disadvantage and have to make additional efforts if their instructions are to be followed.

Characteristics of the Regimen

Among the principle factors associated with patient adherence to a therapeutic or preventive regimen are the characteristics of the regimen itself—the type of regimen, the cost factors, degree of behavioral change required, and so on. Table 7-1 summarizes some of the most important of these characteristics and the way in which each is related to adherence. An analysis of thse factors is essential to an understanding of patient adherence to oral health care recommendations.

TABLE 7-1. **Factors Associated with Adherence
to Health Care Regimens**

| | Probability of Adherence | |
	High	Low
Complexity	Regimen is simple, involves behaviors that are pleasant or interesting	Regimen is complex, involves behaviors that are difficult, time-consuming, boring, or unpleasant
Duration	Regimen involves activities that are short-term or infrequent	Regimen is long-term, involves continued performance of behaviors
Patient's Role	Patient assumes a passive role	Patient must play an active role, assume major responsibility for own care
Consequences	Adherence to regimen produces rapid relief from pain or noticeable improvement in symptoms	Adherence to regimen produces unpleasant side effects; no short-term benefits are apparent

Complexity.   On the surface, the behaviors that we instruct our patients to perform appear very simple. But are they? Good motor-skill performance depends to a great extent on feedback about the accuracy of one's performance. Imagine trying to reproduce a design or drawing if your hand was shielded so that you could not see the results of your efforts. In many ways, we give a similar task to our patients—to reach into a "darkened, inaccessible labyrinth,"[18] cleanse it, and then assess the results of their efforts.

Home care procedures are also time-consuming. Although patients agree that 5 to 8 minutes daily is not an unreasonable amount of time to spend on oral hygiene activities, very few actually spend more than a small fraction of that time. Even among dental students, a group from whom we would expect conscientious oral hygiene practices, a total of 45 seconds has been calculated as the average amount of time spent cleaning the oral cavity.[19] In a study of patient brushing behavior, similar results were obtained.[20] Patients were told that they were participating in a "toothpaste study" in order to disguise the nature of the study. When given a brush and paste and asked to brush as they usually did, patients were observed to brush an average of less than 1 minute. Although these patients reported that they brushed for the same amount of time during the study as at home, they estimated their usual brushing time as 2½ minutes—more than twice as long as they were actually observed to brush. Thus, patients often overestimate the amount of time they spend cleaning their teeth—a fact which might help to explain why some patients stoutly maintain, "I'm doing just what you told me to do," in spite of evidence to the contrary.

Overestimation of time spent brushing and flossing can be explained, in part, by the fact that these are not especially exciting activities. As one writer has observed, "If periodontal disease were controlled by placing electrodes on the teeth with lead wires connected to a device with many dials, blinking red lights, and an oscilloscope or two, control programs would be downright interesting and might even result in a club or association being formed akin to that of the CB radio following."[18] As we know, this is not the case. Oral health care activities remain chores—necessary, but not much fun.

Duration.   It is usually not difficult to persuade patients to adhere to a regimen that lasts only for a brief period of time or one that requires only occasional, infrequent bursts of effort. Most patients, for example, are willing to receive an innoculation to prevent contagious disease. Unfortunately, we do not have a procedure comparable to the innoculation available at this time in the area of oral health care. Good oral health requires a daily program of plaque removal, not just for a week or even a month, but through an entire lifetime.

The patient's role.   As Weinstein points out, there are 8760 hours in a year, of which only a very few are spent with the dentist or physician.[21] It is obvious that prevention cannot be accomplished solely through professional care: Patients must assume active, responsible roles in their own oral health care.

Sadly, many people have become accustomed to thinking of health care as something provided for them by experts. They view their own roles as passive and believe that it is the expert's responsibility to take care of them. When recommendations are made for such professionally provided services as cleaning and application of topical fluoride treatments and occlusal surface sealants, patients are often willing to comply. In fact, research shows that people are considerably more likely to follow recommendations for self-care activities that involve clinic care than they are to follow recommendations that involve self-care only. In a study comparing participation in two preventive programs, children who received professionally delivered topical treatments were twice as likely as children who participated in an at-home mouthrinse program to remain in the program until its completion.[22]

Consequences.   When the consequences of adhering, or failing to adhere, to a health care regimen are readily felt or seen by the patient, the probability of adherence is greatly increased. Conversely, adherence is less likely when the consequences are long-range and/or uncertain. This is true not only for adherence behavior, but for all human behavior. As the work of Harvard psychologist B. F. Skinner and others has shown, behavior tends to be most strongly influenced by consequences that immediately follow the behavior.

When negative or punishing consequences follow a behavior, the behavior is less likely to occur again. For example, if you put your hand on a hot stove and suffer a painful burn as a result, you will be less likely to touch hot stoves in the future. Positive or rewarding consequences, on the other hand, tend to strengthen behavior, making it more likely to be repeated. Behavior is most likely to be repeated when consequences for the behavior are *positive, immediate*, and *certain*.

Thus, when medication provides relief from painful or distressing symptoms, patients are more likely to take it as prescribed than they are when it is taken prophylactically or for symptoms that the patient cannot easily detect. There is a high rate of nonadherence associated with asymptomatic diseases such as hypertension. Similarly, patients often discontinue antibiotic therapy prematurely because symptoms of the infection have abated.

Even when the consequences of nonadherence are unpleasant or actually dangerous, a delay between the behavior and its consequences can seriously affect adherence. The delay need not be lengthy; among dialysis patients, for example, a period of only a day or so between nonadherence and subsequent painful consequences is sufficient to reduce adherence to food and fluid regimens.

When we analyze preventive oral hygiene behavior in terms of consequences, it is apparent that there are few immediate positive consequences for adhering to a preventive regimen. In addition, negative consequences that result from failure to adhere are not obvious to the patient for some time, as caries and periodontal disease develop slowly and present no distressing symptoms until the disease state is quite advanced.

In summary, then, patients fail to adhere to health care recommendations for many reasons other than simply "uncooperative personalities." Many factors influence the likelihood that a patient will be conscientious in following recommendations for preventive home care. Although many of these factors lie outside the control of the health care professional, some can be influenced or altered by the professional. In the next chapter, we will describe some ways in which the oral health professional can help patients acquire more beneficial oral health habits.

REFERENCES

1. National Dairy Council. Nutrition and oral health. *Dairy Council Digest* 49:13, 1978.

2. Young, W., Striggler, D., and Russell, A. *The dentist, his practice, and his community.* Philadelphia: W.B. Saunders Co., 1969.

3. Katz, S., McDonald, J.L., and Stookey, G.K. *Preventive dentistry in action.* Montclair, N.J.: D.C.P. Publishing, 1976.

4. American Dental Association, Bureau of Economic and Behavioral Research. Dental habits and opinions of the public: Results of a 1978 survey. Chicago: American Dental Association, 1979.

5. National Center for Health Statistics. Current estimates from the Health Interview Survey, United States—1978. Series 10, No. 130. Washington, D.C.: U.S. Government Printing Office, 1979.

6. Craig, T., and Montague, J.L. Family and oral health survey. *Journal of the American Dental Association* 92:326, 1976.

7. Ingersoll, B.D., Ingersoll, T.G., McCutcheon, W.R., and Seime, R.J. Behavioral dimensions of dental practice: A national survey. Unpublished manuscript, West Virginia University School of Dentistry, 1979.

8. Sackett, D.L. The magnitude of compliance and noncompliance. In *Compliance with therapeutic regimens*, edited by D.L. Sackett and R.B. Haynes. Baltimore, Md.: Johns Hopkins University Press, 1976.

9. Davis, M.S. Variations in patients' compliance with doctors' orders: Analysis of congruence between survey responses and results of empirical investigations. *Journal of Medical Education* 41:1037, 1966.

10. Haynes, R.B. A critical review of the "determinants" of patient compliance with therapeutic regimens. In *Compliance with therapeutic regimens*, edited by D.L. Sackett and R.B. Haynes. Baltimore, Md.: Johns Hopkins University Press, 1976.

11. Kreisberg, L., and Treiman, B.R. Socioeconomic status and utilization of dentists' services. *Journal of the American College of Dentistry* 27:147, 1960.

12. Nikias, M.K. Social class and use of dental care under prepayment. *Medical Care* 6:381, 1968.

13. Becker, M.H., and Maiman, L.A. Sociobehavioral determinants of compliance with health and medical care recommendations. *Medical Care* 13:10, 1975.

14. Kegeles, S.S. Why people seek dental care: A test of a conceptual formulation. *Journal of Health and Human Behavior* 4:166, 1963.

15. Francis, V., Korsch, B.M., and Morris, M.J. Gaps in doctor-patient communications. *New England Journal of Medicine* 280:535, 1969.

16. Crisci, R., and Kassinove, H. Effect of perceived expertise, strength of advice and environmental setting on parental compliance. *Journal of Social Psychology* 89:245, 1973.

17. Levine, B.A., Moss, K.C., Ramsey, P.H., and Fleishman, R.A. Patient compliance with advice as a function of communicator expertise. *Journal of Social Psychology* 104:309, 1978.

18. Derbyshire, J.C. Motivation of patients. In *Periodontal therapy*, edited by H.M. Goldman and D.W. Cohen. St. Louis, Mo.: C.V. Mosby, 1968.

19. Editorial. The ineffective toothbrush. *Lancet* 2:42, 1960.

20. Yankell, S.L., Emling, R., and Flickinger, K. Patient perception of brushing time compared to actual brushing time, age, and dental care. Paper presented at the meeting of the International Association for Dental Research, Chicago, March, 1981.

21. Weinstein, P. Behavioral strategies to enhance patient compliance with preventive recommendations. In *Advances in behavioral research in dentistry*, edited by P. Weinstein. Seattle: University of Washington, 1978.

22. Lund, A.K., Kegeles, S.S., and Weisenberg, M. Motivational techniques for increasing acceptance of preventive health measures. *Medical Care* 15:678, 1977.

8

Improving Adherence

How can we persuade people to take a more active, responsible role in their own health care? If we were to approach a large group of oral health professionals and ask this question, we would probably receive a variety of responses. "Educate them," some would suggest, while others would respond, "Scare them." Some would say, "Punish them for non-adherence," and still others might suggest, "Reward them when they adhere." All of these approaches have been employed, with varying degrees of success. In the following sections, we will discuss these approaches, as well as others that have been used in the ongoing struggle to persuade patients to do what is best for themselves.

EDUCATIONAL APPROACHES

The assumption underlying the educational approach is that people tend to behave rationally and that if they are given accurate information, they will generally adopt a wise course of action. As quite a bit of research has shown, this assumption is probably untenable, at least with regard to preventive health care behavior. Study after study has demonstrated the ineffectiveness of campaigns urging people to stop smoking, control their weight, exercise regularly, eat nutritious foods, and wear seat belts.

Educational approaches aimed at promoting better oral health behavior have fared no better. In one recent survey, for example, over 40 percent of those questioned reported that instructions alone had no effect whatsoever on their subsequent oral hygiene behavior.[1]

The failure of numerous information programs designed to teach people the facts about dental disease and to alert them to the need for preventive activities has led some investigators to use "fear appeals." This approach emphasizes the painful and distressing results of dental neglect in an attempt to frighten people into following preventive recommendations. Results of this approach have been disappointing. Researchers have discovered that people simply "tune out" messages in which the level of fear is very high (when, for example, they are shown gory pictures of patients with advanced oral disease). When moderate or low fear messages are used in an attempt to persuade, there is no evidence of greater improvement in preventive behavior than is obtained with simple informational messages.[2]

Other investigators have hypothesized that changing the habits of children might prove easier than changing the habits of adults, and that habits, once acquired, would persist as the child matured. This belief has fostered several large-scale preventive programs aimed at school children, such as the Toothkeeper and Toothtown programs.[3,4] Results of these programs, unfortunately, have been all too similar to the results obtained with adults: Although some of them have produced increases in knowledge, positive changes in attitudes toward oral health, and even short-term improvement in preventive behavior, none has succeeded in bringing about the long-term improvement in preventive behavior necessary for the prevention of oral disease.

One writer has summarized the disappointing results of educational/informational programs as follows:

> There is no objective evidence that dental health educational programs to change behavior of individuals with regard to oral hygiene have been effective. . . . Knowing does not mean that doing will follow. Almost everyone knows about the importance of oral hygiene, avoiding sweets and regular visits to the dentist. A great deal of evidence, however, indicates that these behaviors are not enacted, or are inconsistent and inefficient at best.[5]

What are the implications of these findings for the clinician? Do they mean that practitioners should no longer bother to provide patients with information about oral disease and preventive measures? We do *not* mean to imply that this is the case. Certainly, patients need information about the etiology and sequelae of dental caries and periodontal disease. They also need to be made aware of their own vulnerability to these diseases. But patients need more than information and intellectual understanding. They need skill training, and they need assistance in developing new habit patterns. In short, patients need help in changing their *behavior.* We will focus on these points in the following sections.

INITIATING BEHAVIOR CHANGE

Brushing and flossing, like all motor behaviors, require a certain amount of skill if they are to produce the desired results. For many adult patients, of course, the problem lies not in the lack of the requisite skills, but in failure to use these skills on a regular basis. Nevertheless, it is unwise to assume that a patient knows how to brush and floss correctly. It is much safer to ask the patient to demonstrate the technique for you. If the skills are deficient, a training program is in order.

Skills Training

A good program for teaching brushing and flossing should begin with a *demonstration* of the proper technique. We know that people learn most efficiently when they are shown, rather than simply told, what to do. It is also useful to demonstrate some common errors to help the patient learn to discriminate between the correct technique and incorrect methods, because all motor-skill learning involves learning to distinguish between correct and incorrect approaches.

Supervised practice with immediate feedback is also essential to the acquisition of effective motor skills. Disclosing tablets are an excellent means of providing patients with immediate visual feedback about the adequacy of their efforts. Of course, many dental professionals are aware of this and routinely use disclosing agents as part of in-office teaching and to facilitate home practice.

In addition to visual cues, other sensory cues can be helpful in learning brushing and flossing skills. Most adult patients can discriminate between the taste of a clean mouth and one that has not been cleaned adequately. Since the use of flavored toothpaste can mask or obscure these cues and provide the sensation of a clean mouth even when brushing and flossing have not been thorough, some dental professionals recommend that patients be taught to brush using only a brush and water at first. When the patient can achieve the taste and sensation of a clean mouth using only these tools and dental floss, he can then "graduate" to the use of toothpaste.

Establishing Goals

When the patient can demonstrate the ability to achieve a clean mouth in the office, under your supervision, the next step is to establish a regimen of home care activities and preventive visits. Common sense and respect for your patients dictate that this regimen be negotiated between you and the patient, rather than simply imposed on the patient; most people are more receptive to recommendations when they are made to feel a part of the planning process. The following suggestions are intended as a guide for presenting your recommendations to patients:

1. Present your recommendations: "Mrs. Smith, you've mastered the skills necessary to take care of your mouth properly. In order to take the best possible care of your oral health, I suggest the following." (Make specific recommendations concerning frequency of recall visits, and frequency and duration of home care activities.)

2. Ask for feedback: "How does this sound to you?"

In response to this question, the patient will probably either agree to comply with your recommendations (in this case, you should proceed to Step 3) or offer a protest. Most commonly, the protest concerns the amount of time and effort required: "That's an awful lot of toothbrushing!" or "How am I supposed to find the time to do all that?"

It is tempting, of course, to respond to these and similar protests by pointing out that the time spent on oral health care is really minimal in relation to the benefits the patient will reap in the long run. If you think about it for a moment though, you will realize that such a response ignores the patient's feelings and amounts to little more than arguing with him. Remember, "negotiate" does not mean "debate."

Helpful responses include those that evidence recognition of the patient's feelings. You might say, for example: "It sounds like you think I'm being too demanding—that perhaps I don't understand your busy schedule" or "It does sound like a lot of time and effort. You wonder if it's really worth it."

If the patient perceives you as supportive and understanding of his point of view, he will often give up his protests as unnecessary and get down to the business of negotiating a mutually agreeable regimen. At this point, you can offer your assistance in helping him fit the regimen into his schedule.

But what about the patient who announces that he simply is not interested in investing time, effort, and money in caring for his oral health? "Look, I really don't want to be bothered. My sister spent a fortune running around to dentists and still wound up with false teeth. It's just not worth the trouble to me."

Again, it is tempting to argue with this patient, to try to persuade him to see things your way. If you have already explained the consequences of neglect to the patient, however, any additional attempts will usually be futile and will probably just serve to antagonize the patient. It is, after all, the patient's decision—whether you agree with it or not.

What, then, can you do? Your decision will reflect office policy. Some practitioners refuse to treat patients who do not maintain acceptable levels of oral hygiene. For instance, one successful dentist makes a contractual agreement with every new patient. According to the terms of the contract, he will begin treatment only when the patient has reached a certain level of oral hygiene. The dentist reports that it is the rare patient who fails to live up to the contract.

Other dentists offer alternatives to such patients, like more frequent recall visits for patients whose home care practices result in unacceptable levels of cleanliness. (The problem with this strategy, of course, is that patients who lack sufficient motivation and interest to engage in good home care are not likely to follow through with frequent recall visits.) Still others are willing to accept the patient's decision and to lower their own expectations for such patients. They console themselves with the knowledge that they are at least doing what they can for these patients and with the hope that some of them will eventually improve.

3. Write a contract. When you have negotiated a satisfactory agreement with the patient, your task is not finished until you have put the agreement in writing. Written contracts between patient and provider can improve patient adherence to preventive regimens, in part because they help to ensure that the patient won't forget the instructions. Research indicates that patients who can recall their physician's instructions with complete accuracy are three times more likely to comply with the instructions than are patients who make one or more errors in recalling the instructions.[6] Unfortunately, the speed with which patients forget instructions is little short of astonishing. In one large study, investigators found that within a few minutes to an hour or so after leaving the physician's office, patients remembered only a little more than half of what they had been told.[7]

Written instructions concerning the agreed-upon regimen also emphasize to the patient that you consider the regimen important. We know that patients often view health care instructions and advice as less important than other kinds of health care information. When providers take special pains to stress the importance of instructions and recommendations, patient recall improves.[8]

When both patient and provider *sign* the agreement, the agreement is elevated to the status of a contract. By tradition in our society, greater psychological weight or importance is usually accorded to a written contract which both parties have signed than to simple verbal agreements.

Contracts between patient and provider should be quite specific as to the behaviors expected of the patient. In turn, the patient should know exactly what to expect from the provider. A contract that states the services to be provided implies a partnership and shared responsibility for maintaining good oral health. Contracts can also include specific consequences for behavior. These contracts, known as contingency contracts, are discussed in the next section.

THE USE OF CUES AND CONSEQUENCES TO IMPROVE HOME CARE

We have noted that patients often protest about the time required for home care activities. In fact, one of the most common reasons patients give for failure to adhere to a regimen they have agreed to follow is, "I couldn't seem to find the time." A closer analysis often reveals that the problem is one of *poor timing*, rather than the *amount of time* required. Careful selection of times to be set aside for home care activities is a critical ingredient of a successful preventive program. Unless specific times during the day are established as part of the contract negotiated with the patient, it is likely that oral health activities will be shunted aside by competing activities and forgotten, despite the patient's best intentions.

To help patients remember that "This is the time to clean my teeth," we can use a variety of reminders, or *cues.* Artificial cues, such as signs or notices posted in conspicuous places in the patient's home or office, can serve as helpful reminders.

It is even more effective, however, to use naturally occurring cues. This can be done by associating oral health activities with some other fixed activity or event in the patient's daily life, such as watching the evening news or taking a shower. Linking a desired behavior with one that is already a well-established habit increases the likelihood that the desired behavior will itself become a habit.

We can increase the probability of habit formation even more by linking the new behavior and the established habit in such a fashion that the new behavior is performed before the habit. For example, the patient who takes a shower each morning can be instructed to brush and floss before showering. Similarly, a patient whose daily routine includes removing her makeup at bedtime can be encouraged to care for her teeth before removing her makeup. In this way, the opportunity to engage in the habitual behavior can serve as a reward for oral hygiene behavior.

As numerous psychological experiments have demonstrated, consequences that follow a particular behavior have a powerful effect on the likelihood that the behavior will be repeated. Behavior change is facilitated when consequences are positive (rewarding), immediate, and certain—that is, when there is an immediate payoff for performing the behavior. Unfortunately, the negative consequences of dental neglect are long-range, while there are few naturally occurring positive consequences that immediately follow the performance of oral hygiene behaviors.

Behavioral scientists have sought to encourage good oral health habits by rearranging environmental consequences so that immediate positive consequences (rewards) are made to follow desired oral hygiene behaviors. Programs employing the systematic use of rewards for preventive activities have produced promising results in a variety of settings. Several such programs have been conducted with children in the school setting. In some, children received small prizes for brushing or engaging in other targeted preventive behaviors, such as using an acidulated phosphate mouthrinse.[9,10] One innovative group of researchers obtained excellent results simply by posting the child's photograph on a bulletin board as a reward for careful brushing. Children who were rewarded in this fashion showed marked reductions in plaque counts.[11]

Reward programs have also been used successfully in other group settings. For example, when swimming was used as a reward for brushing in a summer camp for boys, the rate of daily brushing increased from about zero to almost 100 percent.[12] Other studies have shown that reward programs can be used to improve oral hygiene behavior among elderly residents in a nursing home and to motivate institutional staff to provide daily toothbrushing for residents unable to perform the task for themselves.[13,14]

In general, then, there is considerable evidence that carefully planned reward programs are an effective method for improving preventive oral health behavior. That dental professionals recognize the importance of rewards—at least with children—is suggested by the time-honored practice of giving a small prize or trinket at the end of the visit. This prize is usually given noncontingently, however; that is, the prize is given regardless of the child's behavior. It is a gift rather than a reward, and it is therefore unlikely to have marked effects on the child's dental behavior either in the office or at home. This is not to say that this practice should be discontinued. Research shows that children view these gifts with enthusiasm and suggests that gift-giving probably helps promote positive feelings about the dental visit.[15] Rather, we urge that in addition to the traditional end-of-the-visit gift you also make systematic use of rewards to encourage desirable behavior.

Reward Programs with Child Patients

Reward programs for children need not be complicated or expensive. Children are pleased with inexpensive trinkets, and young children particularly enjoy the excitement of reaching into a "grab bag" to retrieve a small prize. Other rewards for lowered plaque scores include trophies, wallet cards, and club memberships. Public posting of the child's photograph, found to be effective in the school setting, can also be used in the dental setting.

You might also consider implementing a "double-barrel" approach that combines the opportunity to earn rewards with the use of a color-coded graph such as we have used in our clinic to provide feedback to parents (see next section). The color-coded graph, which can be made from construction paper, consists of a green band covering plaque scores in the "good" range (80 to 100 percent plaque-free surfaces), a yellow band covering the "caution" range (50 to 79 percent plaque-free surfaces), and a red band indicating the "danger" zone (0 to 49 percent plaque-free surfaces). According to this method, the child whose plaque score falls in the red "danger" zone will earn only a single end-of-the-visit prize, but he can earn two prizes if his score falls in the yellow "caution" range, and three prizes for a score in the green "good" range.

Children can also be taught to keep daily records of brushing and flossing. They should be encouraged to bring these records to each dental appointment. The simple act of observing and recording one's own behavior can often stimulate behavior change. In one study, for example, children were given a chart and directions for recording the number of times they brushed each day.[16] The number of times these children brushed daily was significantly higher than the brushing frequency was in a control group of children who were given similar oral hygiene instructions but who were not given the opportunity to chart their behavior.

A sample chart for home recording is given in Figure 8-1. When you instruct the child in the use of the chart, it is also a good idea to provide colorful stars or stickers to be placed on the chart each time he brushes—a simple and inexpensive way to give a reward immediately following each instance of the desired behavior.

So far, the reward programs we have described have all used tangible rewards. It is very important to remember that other kinds of rewards can serve as well, or even better, to strengthen behavior. When you smile at a patient and say enthusiastically, "You've really done a great job!" you are providing a *social reward.* Social rewards are signs of approval, attention, and interest, such as smiles, winks, hugs, and praise.

Whenever a material reward is given, it should always be accompanied by a social reward. It also helps to let your child patient over-

Week	Monday	Tuesday	Wednesday	Thursday	Friday	Saturday	Sunday
1							
2							
3							
4							

Figure 8-1 Sample chart for home recording

hear you praising his performance to someone else—the dentist, for example, or the child's parents. A compliment given in front of another person is especially rewarding.

We have discussed a variety of ways in which reward programs can be used with children in the dental office. The effectiveness of a reward program conducted by the dental professional is somewhat limited, however, because contact with the child is infrequent. You will probably be most effective if, in addition to providing an in-office reward program, you also spend some time teaching parents how to set up and use reward programs in the home.

A great deal of research evidence indicates that parents can be taught to use this approach effectively. For example, Talsma describes a simple but effective reward program used to encourage morning toothbrushing in an 11-year-old boy who regularly brushed on his own initiative at night but seldom, if ever, in the morning.[17] The boy expressed an interest in adding to his coin collection, so seven inexpensive coins he selected were purchased (total cost $2.35), to be used as rewards for morning brushing. The coins were arranged in order of value so that the least valuable coin required the least effort: Only a single morning brushing was sufficient to earn this coin. The second coin required two additional consecutive days of morning brushing; the third, three additional consecutive days, and so on. Each coin was awarded immediately after the necessary number of brushings had occurred. In addition to these tangible rewards, family members expressed interest in the child's progress and praised him for success. This program resulted in an immediate change from no morning brushings to a perfect rate of daily morning brushings for 28 consecutive days. The coin rewards were discontinued after the twenty-eighth day, but the family continued to provide occasional praise for good performance, and the boy continued to brush regularly in the morning on his own initiative.

This case report illustrates several features that should be incorporated into the design of an at-home reward program:

> *Rewards used were items valued by the child.* Obviously, a reward that is not valued by the recipient will do little to promote behavior change. To ensure that the rewards used are valued by the child, involve the child in selecting the rewards. Some negotiation will probably be necessary, especially if the child initially insists that he is only willing to work to earn a pony or a motorcycle or some other reward the parents consider inappropriate or too expensive. It is not wise to argue with the child on this point. Instead, the parent should just arrange other rewards the child is sure to enjoy and then announce the availability of these rewards for performing the desired behavior. If the rewards have been selected

carefully, the child's initial protests will quickly fade as he works to earn the rewards.

Rewards were delivered immediately after each target behavior was performed. When long delays occur between performance of the behavior and delivery of the reward, the reward's effectiveness is greatly reduced.

Progress toward the long-range goal (regular, independent morning brushings) *was broken into smaller behavioral steps, and each step was rewarded.* At first, rewards were dispensed frequently and required only minimal levels of performance. As the child progressed, the size of the steps increased; rewards required increasing levels of performance and were dispensed less frequently. (Note that this type of program also allows the child to accumulate daily "points" toward a larger or more expensive reward than might be provided on a daily basis. When using a program like this, it is a good idea to include additional smaller rewards at shorter intervals so the child does not become bored or discouraged.)

That these factors are essential to the success of a reward program is nicely illustrated by a study in which an at-home reward program was used to increase the frequency with which a 16-year-old boy wore his orthodontic appliance.[18] After eight years of treatment, the boy showed essentially no change in his orthodontic condition, because he did not wear his headband as prescribed.

In the first phase of this program, the parents made five unannounced observations daily, at varying intervals. At each observation, the parents simply recorded whether or not their son was wearing the appliance. As Table 8-1 shows, the appliance was in place during an average of only 25 percent of the daily observations—far less than the

TABLE 8-1. Results of Several Strategies to Increase Amount
of Time Orthodontic Appliance in Place

Phase	Percent of Observations Device in Place
Baseline (observation only)—8 days	25
Social reward (praise)—9 days	36
Delayed monetary reward/fine—35 days	60
Immediate monetary reward/fine—18 days	97
Post-checks	100

Summarized from R. Hall, S. Axelrod, L. Tyler, E. Grief, F.C. Jones, and R. Robertson. Modification of behavior problems in the home with a parent as an observer and experimenter (*Journal of Applied Behavior Analysis* 5:53, 1972).

amount of time recommended by the orthodontist. During the second phase, the parents praised the boy each time they observed him wearing the appliance but made no comment when the appliance was not in place. This resulted in a slight increase from baseline levels (to 36 percent of observations). Greater improvement was seen in the third phase, when a delayed monetary reward was used; the boy could earn 25 cents each time the appliance was in place during an observation and would be fined 25 cents if the appliance was not in place, but he would neither receive the money nor pay the fines until the end of the month. Although this procedure resulted in an increase in appliance wearing (to 60 percent of observations), a much greater increase (to 97 percent) resulted when an on-the-spot reward/fine policy was implemented in the fourth phase. In the final phase of this program, the parents checked their son at infrequent, irregular intervals and provided an on-the-spot reward or fine for presence or absence of the appliance. This approach resulted in virtually constant wearing of the appliance. Eight months after this reward program was initiated, the orthodontist stated that the boy no longer needed to wear the appliance, as great improvement in his mouth structure had been achieved.

This study also illustrates the importance of weaning a child from a reward program gradually, so that decreases in the frequency of the previously rewarded behavior do not result. When rewards are withdrawn abruptly, the previously rewarded behavior often quickly drops to former low levels. Parents can foresee such a problem, and many worry that they will wind up with 30-year-old sons or daughters who will not brush or floss unless their parents reward them with a quarter.

As the study demonstrates, this need not be the case, so you can reassure parents about this point. Parents should be instructed to continue the reward program until the new behavior is well established (usually a period of several weeks to a few months). They can then begin to phase out rewards gradually, using surprise spot checks. These spot checks should be made every other day or so, then decreased to every 3 or 4 days, and so on until they are no longer necessary.

Other points to remember when helping parents establish reward programs for their children include the following:

Avoid the "material reward trap." Although rewards are not really bribes (the dictionary defines a *bribe* as "anything given to induce a person to do something illegal or wrong"), many parents are nevertheless uncomfortable with the notion of providing tangible rewards to help their children learn new behaviors. In addition, the cost of a reward program using only material rewards can add up quickly, even if relatively inexpensive rewards are used. Instead of relying solely on material rewards, parents should be encouraged to use *activity rewards.* Activity rewards include any activity the child enjoys, such as watching television, playing a game, riding a bike, staying up past bedtime, and having a friend spend the night. Activity rewards need not be special events, although special events can easily be used as rewards simply by allowing the child to earn points toward the activity. Of course, parents should also be reminded to use social rewards very frequently. No child has ever suffered ill effects from too much praise for good behavior.

Use a variety of rewards. To avoid a situation in which the child becomes bored with a particular reward, it is a good idea to provide a variety of rewards. Children can help construct a "reward menu" or, with younger children, a grab bag can be used to provide variety and excitement.

Reward Programs with Adult Patients

It requires only a moment's thought to realize that developing effective reward programs for adult patients is, in many ways, very different from using rewards with children. Most adults are less than enthusiastic at the prospect of earning balloons and gold stars or having their pictures posted on your bulletin board. An additional distinguishing point is that with children, the parents can serve as agents of reward for good behavior in the home. The adult, on the other hand, must serve as his own rewarding agent.

Research and clinical experience have shown that reward programs that are self-administered can be very effective in promoting behavior change and in maintaining behavior. Most of us, in fact, use self-rewards far more than we might realize. Such self-administered rewards as telling ourselves, "I did a good job," or "I'll read one more chapter in this textbook and then I'll have a snack," are probably essential for maintaining many of our everyday behaviors.

Patients can be helped to set up their own self-administered reward programs whereby they systematically reward themselves with a favorite activity or a tangible reward for brushing and flossing. A patient might decide, for example, that he will watch the evening news only if he has carefully brushed and flossed first. Another patient might decide that treating herself to lunch at a favorite restaurant would be an enticing reward for one full week of good home care. Many useful suggestions for implementing self-reward programs can be found in Weinstein and Getz's interesting book, *Changing Human Behavior: Strategies for Preventive Dentistry.* *

When the patient has decided upon a suitable set of goals and re-

*Chicago: SRA, 1978.

wards, the details of the program should be specified in a patient-provider contract in the following form:

I ___(Patient)___ will do the following ___(Specific behavior)___

in return for ___(Reward)___ .

Signed ___(Patient)___

Signed ___(Provider)___

Date _____

Note that the wording of this simple contract is positive in tone. Avoid contracts that are negatively stated and involve punishing consequences. "If I brush and floss, I will reward myself by watching the news" is better than "If I don't brush and floss, I can't watch the news." Since our goal is to strengthen desirable behavior by associating the behavior with pleasurable consequences, we should be sure to emphasize rewards and success instead of punishment and failure.

Contracts such as the one above, which specify behaviors to be performed and the consequences that will follow the behaviors, are called *contingency contracts.* In health care programs, contingency contracts have been used successfully to help obese patients lose weight[19] and to control drug abuse.[20] In one study using contingency contracting with hypertensive patients, patients in the contracting group acquired significantly more knowledge about hypertension and remained in clinic care longer than did patients who did not participate in contracting.[21] Further, blood pressures for patients in the contracting group quickly dropped to levels considered "under control" and remained there, while pressures for patients who did not contract fluctuated considerably.

Contingency contracts that involve the dental professional as a source of tangible rewards have also been used with success. In one very interesting study, patients in a private periodontal practice contracted for fee reductions based on their plaque scores at the last of three visits.[22] For patients whose plaque scores were 20 percent or less at the final visit, the total fee was reduced by 10 percent. A final plaque score of 10 percent or less resulted in a fee reduction of 25 percent. Results of this study indicated significantly greater reductions in plaque scores among contract patients than among patients who went through an identical educational program but who were not offered an opportunity to contract. At the 6-month recall visit, the contract group had maintained these gains.

While this study demonstrates that fee-based contingency contracts can be a very effective means of improving oral hygiene behavior, we must ask whether such an approach is economically feasible. Addressing this question, the authors of the study point out that many patients who otherwise would not participate in a preventive program might be motivated by such a contract to participate, thus increasing the total number of patients treated in the practice. In addition, fees and refund schedules could be adjusted to promote participation without sacrificing cost-efficiency.

Finally, do not overlook the power of social rewards. Patients are very sensitive to praise and criticism—so much so, in fact, that some patients avoid the dental office because they fear being belittled or scolded for the condition of their mouths. Be generous, then, in your use of social rewards. Although we all enjoy receiving praise for our efforts, most of us are surprisingly stingy in dispensing it to others. In fact, if you were actually to count and record the number of times in an average working day that you complimented a patient, it is likely that the total would be much lower than you might think.

Try this simple little experiment to check yourself and, at the same time, improve your skills. Use an index card or a golf-stroke counter to record each time you praise a patient for some aspect of his performance. Keep a record for a week and determine your average daily rate. Then, for the second week, set a figure slightly higher than this average as a goal to be reached each day. Since your performance is more likely to improve if positive consequences follow your behavior, rearrange events in your schedule to provide small rewards for improvement. Coffee breaks or a special treat at lunch could be used as rewarding consequences. Or you might set aside a small sum of money on each day that you reach your goal. At the end of the week, use this money to buy yourself a treat.

SCHEDULING RECALL VISITS

Frequent recall visits are helpful when patients are attempting to develop new health habits, because they provide an opportunity for patients to receive feedback concerning their progress. We have seen that feedback is important while the patient is attempting to master specific skills; feedback is also useful in helping the patient develop new habit patterns involving the use of these skills. For example, graphing plaque and gingival indexes at each visit provides patients with feedback about their progress and results in significantly lower scores when these patients are compared with patients who do not view graphs of their progress. In an evaluation of the merits of this strategy, three groups of adult patients were compared.[23] One group received only oral physiotherapy instructions, while a second group received instructions and disclosing tablets for at-home use. In addition to instructions and disclosing tablets, a third group were also shown graphs of their gingival and plaque indexes at each visit. Patients in the latter group had significantly lower scores than patients in either of the other groups did at a 10-week follow-up visit. In turn, the scores of the patients who were given disclosing tablets were superior to those of patients who received only instructions. These results support the routine use of disclosing tablets and graphs of plaque and gingival indexes—especially because, as the authors note, plaque and gingival indexes can be made in 2 minutes.

A similar study conducted in our clinic suggests that graphs are also a useful means of improving parents' care of their preschool children's teeth.[24] Color-coded graphs were used, with a green band covering scores in the "good" range (80 to 100 percent plaque-free surfaces); a yellow band covering scores in the "caution" range (50 to 79 percent plaque-free surfaces); and a red band indicating the "danger" zone (0 to 49 percent plaque-free surfaces). All children whose parents were given graphic feedback showed steady improvement in plaque scores across visits. In contrast, performance was very inconsistent in a second group, who were only told their child's score and did not view the color-coded graph. By the fourth visit, the difference between groups was large and statistically significant, indicating the effectiveness of this method for improving oral hygiene performance.

Visual feedback, then, is a simple but effective method for helping patients improve their oral hygiene. Ordinary graph paper can be used for this purpose or, for added impact, a color-coded graph can be made from construction paper. A single graph can show progress over many visits, providing both you and the patient with valuable information at a glance.

Although we have stressed the need for frequent recall appointments to help patients develop good self-care habits, we must also acknowledge that persuading patients to schedule and keep recall appointments is not always easy. The use of a contract helps, as the contract specifies the intervals at which recall visits will occur.

Because patients who leave the office with a vague promise to call later for an appointment show an uncanny knack for "forgetting" to call, it is wise to encourage the patient to schedule his next appointment before he leaves the office. Your choice of words in this situation is important; if you ask the patient, "Would you like to schedule another appointment now?" you are offering him an opportunity to say no. It is preferable to ask, "*When* would you like to schedule your next appointment? What day of the week is most convenient for you?" This approach still leaves the patient free to exercise choice, but it limits his choice to *when* he will come, instead of *whether* he will come.

Of course, scheduling the return appointment successfully does not guarantee that the patient will actually keep the appointment. Broken or cancelled appointments are a very common problem in dentistry. In fact, broken appointment rates are generally reported to be more than 20 percent and can run as high as 50 percent.[25] Broken appointments wreak havoc with a carefully planned office schedule, and every broken appointment represents income lost to the provider.

It is common practice to use reminder notes and reminder telephone calls to encourage patients to keep their appointments. As these methods involve the expenditure of time and money, it is worthwhile to ask whether they are effective in reducing the rate of cancelled and broken appointments. Results of one study in which these methods were evaluated indicated that telephone reminders decreased the rate of broken appointments by 20 percent and postcard reminders decreased the rate by 30 percent.[26] Neither of these methods, however, was as effective as a third strategy: asking patients to call to confirm their appointments. The receptionist gave each patient a reminder card listing instructions to call the clinic to confirm appointments. She also asked each patient to call, which added a more personal touch than the written instructions alone. This method reduced the rate of broken appointments by 60 percent—more than half—and without the extra costs in time and money incurred with the other methods.

It is notable that among patients who called to confirm, almost all (98 percent) kept their appointments. The broken appointments were almost exclusively in the group that did not call to confirm. Thus, we can speculate that the rate of broken appointments might have been reduced still further if the receptionist had called the nonconfirmers to remind them of their appointments.

This method clearly yields excellent results. It is also easy and inexpensive to implement in the dental office, and it requires neither special training nor special materials. Should you consider using it in your office, remember to designate a time by which patients should call to confirm, and have the receptionist personally ask each patient to call the office.

REFERENCES

1. Craig, T., and Montague, J.L. Family and oral health survey. *Journal of the American Dental Association* 92:326, 1976.

2. Leventhal, H. Fear appeals and persuasion: The differentiation of a motivational construct. *American Journal of Public Health* 61:1208, 1971.

3. Masters, D.H. The classroom teacher . . . effective dental health educator. *Journal of the American Society of Preventive Dentistry* 2:4, 1972.

4. National Dairy Council. Toothtown U.S.A., Program description and unit outline. Chicago, 1975.

5. Frazier, P.J. A new look at dental health education in community programs. *Dental Hygiene* 52:176, 1978.

6. Svarstad, B. Physician–patient communication and patient conformity with medical advice. In *The growth of bureaucratic medicine,* edited by D. Mechanic. New York: John Wiley, 1976.

7. Ley, P., and Spelman, M.S. *Communicating with the patient.* London: Staples Press, 1967.

8. Ley, P. What the patient doesn't remember. *Medical Opinion Review* 1:69, 1966.

9. Lund, A.K., Kegeles, S.S., and Weisenberg, M. Motivational techniques for increasing acceptance of preventive health measures. *Medical Care* 15:678, 1977.

10. Swain, J.J., Allard, G.B., and Holborn, S.W. The good toothbrushing game: A school-based dental hygiene program for increasing the toothbrushing effectiveness of children. *Journal of Applied Behavior Analysis* 15:171, 1982.

11. Blount, R.L., and Stokes, T.F. Promoting effective toothbrushing by elementary school children using contingent public posting of photographs. Poster session presented at the meeting of the Association for the Advancement of Behavior Therapy, Toronto, November, 1981.

12. Lattal, K.A. Contingency management of toothbrushing in a summer camp for children. *Journal of Applied Behavior Analysis* 2:195, 1969.

13. Kiyak, A. An experimental preventive dentistry program for institutionalized elderly. In *Clinical research in behavioral dentistry: Proceedings of the Second National Conference on Behavioral Dentistry,* edited by B. Ingersoll and W. McCutcheon. Morgantown, W.Va.: West Virginia University, 1979.

14. Iwata, B.A., Baily, J.S., Brown, K.M., Foshee, T.J., and Alpern, M. A performance-based lottery to improve residential care and training of institutional staff. *Journal of Applied Behavior Analysis* 9:417, 1976.

15. Morgan, P., Wright, L., Ingersoll, B., and Seime, R. Children's perception of the dental experience. *Journal of Dentistry for Children* 47:243, 1980.

16. Lee, M., McTigue, D., Friedman, C., Carlin, S., Kline, N., and Flintom, C. The visual reinforcement value of a chart on oral hygiene behaviors of children. Paper presented at the meeting of the International Association for Dental Research, Chicago, March, 1981.

17. Talsma, E.M. Contingency management of toothbrushing with an eleven-year-old boy. In *Psychological readings for the dental profession,* edited by B. Van Zoost. Chicago: Nelson-Hall, 1975.

18. Hall, R.V., Axelrod, S., Tyler, L., Grief, E., Jones, F.C., and Robertson, R. Modification of behavior problems in the home with a parent as observer and experimenter. *Journal of Applied Behavior Analysis* 5:53, 1972.

19. Mann, R. The behavior-therapeutic use of contingency contracting to control an adult behavior problem: Weight control. *Journal of Applied Behavior Analysis* 5:99, 1972.

20. Boudin, H.M. Contingency contracting as a therapeutic tool in the deceleration of amphetamine use. *Behavior Therapy* 3:604, 1972.

21. Steckel, S.B., and Swain, M.A. Contracting with patients to improve compliance. *Hospitals* 51:81, 1977.

22. Iwata, B.A., and Becksfort, C.M. Behavioral research in preventive dentistry: Educational and contingency management approaches to the problem of patient compliance. *Journal of Applied Behavior Analysis* 14:111, 1981.

23. Barrickman, R.W., and Penhall, O.J. Graphing indexes reduces plaque. *Journal of the American Dental Association* 87:1404, 1973.

24. Hudock, T., Morgan, M., and Ingersoll, B. Visual feedback to improve parents' care of their preschool children's teeth. Unpublished manuscript, West Virginia University School of Dentistry, 1981.

25. Sackett, D.L. The magnitude of compliance and noncompliance. In *Compliance with therapeutic regimens*, edited by D.L. Sackett and R.B. Haynes. Baltimore, Md.: Johns Hopkins University Press, 1976.

26. Cohen, A. Strategies to reduce broken dental appointments. In *Advances in behavioral research in dentistry*, edited by P. Weinstein. Seattle, Wash.: University of Washington, 1978.

9

The Child Patient

It is a few minutes past five o'clock and Dr. Silver's office is closing for the day. On her way to the door, Dianne Parker, R.D.H., pauses to say good night. Ann, the receptionist, looks up.

"You look beat. Did the kids do you in today?" Ann asks sympathetically.

"Well," Dianne replies, "Cindy and Aaron weren't so bad. In fact, I'd call Aaron a model patient. He doesn't seem at all afraid. He's so relaxed, he almost goes to sleep. He's never a problem. But Jason—now that's another story! Just getting him in the chair wore me out. He cried all the way through the session. I don't think he even stopped to breathe. You'd have thought I was killing him, the way he carried on."

Ann smiles. "Yes, I know. I heard him, and so did everyone else in the office. I'll bet they even heard him out in the hall."

"Yes, and my ear was just 6 inches from his mouth. Boy, do I have a headache," Dianne adds, rubbing her temples.

"Well, go home and put your feet up. You'll have a better day tomorrow."

As the door closes, Ann hears Dianne reply, "Not if we have another one like Jason!"

Why do some children, like Aaron, behave beautifully in the operatory while others, like Jason, make the dental professional long for a quiet job in a boiler factory? How often can you expect to encounter children like Jason? Is there any way to predict how a particular child will react? More importantly, what can be done to prevent or at least minimize behavior that is so distressing to all concerned? We will discuss these questions in the following sections.

INCIDENCE AND ETIOLOGY OF PROBLEM BEHAVIOR

Fortunately for the dental professional, most children do *not* scream, kick, and thrash their way through a visit to the dentist. If you have had much clinical experience with children in the operatory, you know that most children past the age of 4 or 5 years are reasonably cooperative patients. On the other hand, children like the little boy described in the preceding scenario do appear in the dental office with sufficient frequency that in a national survey of practicing dentists, over half of the respondents reported the problem.[1] Studies conducted at the University of Washington revealed that an average of 6 to 7 percent of children seen by general practitioners behave in a problematic way during dental treatment.[2] While this figure might seem inconsequential, it takes on significance when we consider that it means that the average general practitioner can expect to encounter management problems with one to two children each week.

Note the phrase "the *average* general practitioner." These investigators also reported that 15 percent of the dentists they studied described management problems with four or more children each week. Remember, too, that many general-practice dentists refer children with problem behavior to pedodontists, so the incidence of uncooperative children is probably much higher in a pedodontic practice than in a general practice. In fact, almost half of a sample of patients aged 3½ to 9 years drawn from the West Virginia University Pediatric Dental Clinic exhibited 30 percent or more disruptive behavior during restorative treatment—a level of disruptive behavior which over three-quarters of a group of practicing dentists indicated would cause some difficulty in providing safe, high-quality treatment.[3]

The question of why some children behave well during treatment and others do not is especially interesting. There is no simple answer to this question, because many factors determine whether a child will be a calm, cooperative patient or a "holy terror."

Fear and Uncooperative Behavior

Fear is a critical determinant of child behavior, particularly among younger children whose only ways to cope with anxiety are to cry and to try to escape to the safety of the mother's lap. For the child below the age of 3 years, crying and fussing are to be expected when the child is confronted with a situation as strange and overwhelming as the dental visit. As the child matures, negative behavior diminishes, and we can expect increasingly cooperative behavior after about 4 years of age.

There are no sex differences in either cooperative behavior or fearfulness among younger children.[4] As children grow older, girls tend to describe themselves as more fearful than do boys, but there is no evidence to indicate a corresponding increase in uncooperative behavior.[5]

Among elementary-school children, about one-third report some anxiety about dental treatment.[5] Surveys also show that about half this number—roughly 15 to 16 percent—describe themselves as highly fearful. In one survey, for example, when fourth-grade children were asked, "How do you feel in the dentist's chair?" 17 percent of the children in the sample answered by endorsing the response, "I am very scared."[6]

These figures are disturbing because, unlike other childhood fears which are likely to be outgrown as the child matures, dental fear can persist long after the child becomes an adult. It has been reported, for example, that parents (especially mothers) of dentally fearful children had themselves been dentally anxious as children and remained fearful of dentistry as adults.[7] This suggests that dental fear is passed along by example from parents to children, and that anxious children become anxious adults who, in turn, produce dentally fearful offspring.

As we mentioned in our discussion of dental fear in adults, there is considerable evidence to support the idea that unfavorable family attitudes toward dentistry are an important factor in the development of dental fear. When dentally fearful individuals are studied, as many as one-third are found to have had at least one family member who was fearful of dentistry.[8] In keeping with the hypothesis that the mother's attitude is particularly important, many investigators have found a direct relationship between the mother's level of anxiety at her child's first dental visit and the child's anxiety and uncooperative behavior at that visit.[9,10] Of course, when a mother who is herself fearful of dental treatment attempts to prepare her child for the first dental visit, she may do more harm than good. One study showed that when parents attempted to alleviate child anxiety, many children actually became *more* apprehensive.[8]

Another factor which plays a role in the development of fearful responses to dentistry is the child's past experience with physicians.[11] Psychologists use the term *generalization* to describe the process by which something learned in one situation is carried over to other similar situations. The child who has had painful or frightening medical experiences is very likely to generalize the fear of medical personnel and medical treatment to include dental professionals and dental treatment. The situations do, after all, have a great deal in common, including the much-dreaded possibility of "getting a shot."

It is important to emphasize that the relationship between fear and uncooperative behavior during dental treatment, although substantial, is far from direct. Not all uncooperative behavior stems from fear, and not all fearful children are disruptive and uncooperative. Every dental professional has seen children whose behavior could be more appropriately described as "bratty" than fearful. Conversely, it is not uncommon to encounter children who, although obviously very tense, are quiet and cooperative throughout the dental visit.

A case in point from the author's own experience is that of Sarah, a 7-year-old who was observed undergoing restorative treatment. From the start, Sarah's behavior was very subdued, and it was difficult to determine whether she was apprehensive about dental treatment or simply shy in the presence of strangers. Throughout the visit, she showed no obvious signs of resistance or distress, even during the anesthetic injection. Afterward, though, when given a children's picture test and asked to "select the children who feel most like you feel right now," she selected only pictures of children who appeared frightened or unhappy. Then, within a minute of rejoining her parents in the reception area, she fell to the floor in a faint—a dramatic indication of how stressful the experience had been for her.

Unfortunately, the needs of children like Sarah, called *tense-cooperative* children by clinicians, are often overlooked because their behavior does not cause trouble or create difficulty for the dental professional. If the needs of these children do not receive special attention, however, many of them might never overcome their fear of dentistry.

Child Development, Child-Rearing Practices, and Behavior in the Operatory

Normal development.   Most Americans wholeheartedly endorse the belief that "all men are created equal." While all babies may be equal in the eyes of the law, however, they certainly are not all alike, nor do they proceed at identical rates of physical, emotional, and intellectual development.

The child's level of intellectual functioning is an important determinant of the reaction to dental treatment. It is generally agreed that coping with the demands of the dental experience requires a mental age of at least 3 years. Thus, a developmentally delayed child with a chronological age of 4 years but a mental age of only 2 years is likely to be considerably less cooperative than a brighter child who is chronologically younger but who has a mental age of 4 years.

Severe delays in development are usually the result of brain damage associated with such biological abnormalities as chromosomal and metabolic disorders (see Chapter 11). These children often present a distinctive physical appearance, as is the case with Down's syndrome children. Especially in cases of mildly delayed development, however, delayed intellectual functioning is not always readily apparent from the child's physical appearance. Some familiarity with normal patterns of child development can help you know what to expect of children at different ages as well as help you identify children who are developmentally delayed. By spending a few minutes interacting with the child before he enters the operatory, you will have an opportunity to observe the presence or absence of age-appropriate skills and behaviors.

The 2-year-old.   By age two, the average child understands most simple words and sentences. He has a vocabulary of approximately 50 words, uses two- and three-word sentences, and is beginning to use pronouns, although he still refers to himself by name ("Johnny fall down"). He can turn the pages in a book and name familiar items. He has mastered walking, can run fairly well, and can ascend and descend steps alone. Fine motor skills include the ability to imitate a vertical stroke with a crayon and to build a tower of six or seven blocks. As the 2-year-old moves from the dependency of infancy toward increasing competence and independence, he becomes more assertive and experiments with saying no and refusing to do what is asked of him. Frustration at this age is usually expressed physically, with tears and tantrums.

The 3-year-old.   The average 3-year-old has a vocabulary of about 900 words and is able to understand most of the language of ordinary conversation. He refers to himself by pronoun, can describe the action in a picture, and knows a few rhymes or television commercials. He can pedal a tricycle, build a tower of nine to ten blocks, and copy a circle, holding the crayon in his fingers instead of using the entire hand. The competent 3-year-old engages in role-play, let's-pretend, and make-believe. He shows pride in personal accomplishment, seeks approval for activities and achievements, and responds well to praise. Increasing social maturity is evidenced by his ability to take turns and to play in association with other children. Increasing maturity is also seen in his greater control over his own emotions.

The 4-year-old.   By 4 years of age, we expect the child to have mastered a variety of self-help skills, such as dressing and undressing with little assistance, and preparing a bowl of cereal. Fine and gross motor skills continue to develop: The 4-year-old can descend stairs with one foot per tread, push and turn a wagon, copy a cross, and use blocks to build a simple building. Social progress is also evident; the 4-year-old directs an increasing amount of attention toward peers and peer relationships. His play becomes increasingly complex and cooperative. He enjoys dramatic play, such as playing house, store, and hospital, complete with costumes and props. This is the age of which children often have imaginary companions. The 4-year-old enjoys nonsense words, silly language, and rhyming. Emotionally, children of this age tend to be somewhat brash and expansive, with many fluctuations in mood and bursts of strenuous motor activity.

The 5-year-old.   At age five, the child's vocabulary has increased to more than 2000 words, and speech is quite clear. The 5-year-old can copy a triangle, fold a square of paper into a triangle, draw an unmistakable human figure with a body, count ten objects, recognize coins, and copy some numbers. He can also slide down a slide, prepare a sandwich, print his first name, and knows his address. At this age, the child typically enjoys learning to do new things, is willing to accept adult help, and likes to be helpful. In fact, experts in child development have referred to this as "a delightful age" and as "the age of conformity," because 5-year-olds are usually eager to please and concerned with doing the "right thing."[12] Children at this age take special pride in being 5 years old and view themselves as "big boys" and "big girls."

The 6-year-old.   By his sixth birthday, the average child can throw and bounce a ball, skip, and jump rope. Fine motor skills include the ability to tie shoe laces, cut and paste, and draw a human figure with neck, hands, and clothes. At this age, the child is ready to profit from formal instruction in reading, writing, and arithmetic, and can print some words, count 20 objects, and do simple addition and subtraction. He can play simple card games and likes war games, cops and robbers, and cowboys and Indians. This is a period of some variation, and children tend to be somewhat more brash and less generally cooperative than they had been in the preceding year.

The 7-to-12-year-old.   Around the age of seven, important changes occur in the way a child thinks. The child enters what Swiss psychologist Jean Piaget calls *the stage of concrete operations.*[13] By this, Piaget means that the child can think more logically; he can recognize, for example, that when a ball of clay is rolled into a thin rope, the amount of clay remains the same. By this age, the child can pay attention to more cues and can plan before acting, so his behavior is more controlled and inhibited. Fewer brash outbursts occur, and the child is more serious and thoughtful.

The adolescent.   Around the twelfth year, intellectual growth takes another leap as the child moves into *the stage of formal operations.* Prior to this stage, logical reasoning capability is limited to problems involving concrete (actual) objects. In the stage of formal operations, however, the child can handle abstract ideas and hypothetical situations. He can think about concepts like truth, honor, and justice; he develops concern with ideals of conduct, and he can think in terms of the future. The physical changes that occur during this period are often stressful. The hormonal changes of adolescence may be associated with mood swings and mild degrees of hostility, irritability, and anxiety.

Temperament.   Just as children differ in rates of development, so do they differ in personal style, or temperament, as it is called. Some babies are naturally rather placid and easygoing from the start. If a feeding is delayed, a diaper is wet, or some other change in routine occurs, these babies signal their distress with whimpers or quiet cries. In contrast, some babies are much fussier and more intense in their responses. If their needs are not met immediately, they react with screams and howls. Similarly, while some infants are outgoing and respond with eager curiosity to new people, places, and objects, others are more cautious and must be introduced to new situations gradually to avoid tears and protests. And just as some babies quickly fall into a comfortable routine of eating, sleeping, and so on, there are others who are very irregular in their habits and who never seem to settle into a predictable pattern.

These and other facets of child behavior were investigated in a fascinating study in which a large group of children were followed from birth through adolescence.[14] Results of this research revealed that from the earliest weeks and months of life, children show distinctive temperaments that tend to be fairly stable as the child develops. From their observations, the researchers were able to identify three major temperamental styles.

Easy children are generally positive in mood. They are also positive in their approach to new situations and adjust well to change. Regularity in appetite, sleep patterns, and other biological functions simplifies caring for such infants and planning schedules around them. The intensity of their reactions tends to be mild; that is, they are more apt to cry or whimper than shriek, more likely to smile or chuckle than guffaw. When such a child does cry, it is usually a signal that something is indeed amiss.

Difficult children are irregular in biological function, especially in the early months and years of life. Planning routines around these children is problematic. When difficult children encounter new situations—the first bath, a new food, exposure to strangers—they tend to respond with loud protest, withdrawal, or crying. They adapt only slowly. Mood is preponderantly negative; difficult infants tend to cry and fuss more than they laugh. In addition, their reactions are often forceful and intense, and their activity level is high. As we might expect, difficult children are particularly prone to develop behavioral disturbances.

Slow-to-warm-up children share a dislike of change. They respond to new situations with quiet withdrawal, and they are slow to adapt. Activity level is usually low to moderate, responses tend to be mild rather than intense, and if allowed to proceed at their own pace, these children gradually overcome an initial negative response to a new situation and make a good adjustment to it.

What are the implications of these findings for the dental setting? Obviously, temperamentally difficult and slow-to-warm-up children are more apt to pose problems in the operatory than are children who are temperamentally easy (although even easy children can react poorly if they are ill-prepared or harshly treated). With the slow-to-warm-up child, patience combined with the assumption that the child will gradually make a good adjustment will usually produce good results. Greater patience, together with consistent limit setting, will be required with the difficult child.

Child-rearing practices.   A developing child does not exist in a vacuum. Environmental influences, interacting with the child's temperament and other innate endowments, are powerful forces in shaping attitudes and behavior. Among the most important of these environmental influences are the child-rearing practices employed by the parents.

We noted that temperamentally difficult children are particularly prone to develop behavioral disturbances. To a great extent, the outcome with such children depends on how they are reared. If, for example, the parents of a difficult child are intimidated by his stormy tantrums, the child soon learns to rely on shrieks and tantrums to control others. Patience and firm limit setting are needed to help a difficult child learn more acceptable patterns of behavior. While easy children, by definition, pose fewer serious challenges to a parent's child-rearing skills, even an easy child can develop behavior problems as a result of inconsistent disciplinary practices, unrealistic expectations, or a chaotic, stressful environment.

Of particular interest are recent studies focusing on the relationship between child-rearing practices and the way in which children react to medical and dental experiences.[15,16] Results of this research suggest that making appropriate demands on a child and setting clear limits contribute to a child's ability to control his own behavior and to cope with unpleasant situations. If parents are very permissive, set few limits, and seldom discipline, the child is less likely to master these skills.

Concerning the child's reaction to feared situations, in particular, these studies revealed that children whose parents rely on reassurance and rewards for helping them to approach feared situations exhibit more adequate coping behaviors and less anxiety than do children whose parents try to manage these situations using punishment, threats, and force.

Coping behavior in the operatory.   It is clear from the preceding discussion that the complex interaction of many factors determines the manner in which a child react to dental treatment. It is perhaps less obvious (but certainly no less important) that that reaction—whether it be calm and cooperative behavior, shrieks and tears, or white-faced silence—represents *the child's best attempt to cope with a difficult and threatening situation.*

Unlike the adult, who can draw upon skills learned and practiced over many years of dealing with stressful events, the young child has only a limited range of coping skills. Because he has had few opportunities to learn appropriate strategies for coping with unpleasant situations, the inexperienced child patient is likely to resort to such maladaptive strategies as crying, struggling, and attempting to escape.

When we view the situation from this perspective, we can see that our task in pediatric dentistry is not to "manage" the fearful or difficult child but, rather, to help him learn more effective ways to cope. Our goal, then, becomes learning to help the child develop the ability to control himself rather than learning to control the problem child. In the following sections, we will discuss ways to achieve this goal.

ASSESSING AND IMPROVING THE CHILD'S ABILITY TO COPE

Assessment and Prediction of Coping Behavior

Our discussion of the factors that influence a child's ability to adjust to the demands of the dental situation leads to a practical question: From our knowledge of these factors, can we predict which children will cope effectively and which will fail? This question is important because we cannot provide special assistance to children who are limited in their ability to cope unless we can first identify these children. Then, too, it is far more efficient and effective to identify potential problems before the child enters the operatory than to wait until he is screaming hysterically in the chair. The old adage "An ounce of prevention is worth a pound of cure" is particularly apt in the pediatric dental setting.

Much valuable information about the child's ability to make a satisfactory adjustment in the operatory can be obtained from the child's parent, even if the child has never experienced dental treatment. The

	Not afraid at all	A little afraid	A fair amount afraid	Pretty much afraid	Very afraid
1. Dentists					
2. Doctors					
3. Injections (shots)					
4. Having somebody examine your mouth					
5. Having to open your mouth					
6. Having a stranger touch you					
7. Having the nurse clean your teeth					
8. The dentist drilling					
9. Sight of the dentist drilling					
10. Noise of the dentist's drill					
11. Having someone put instruments in your mouth					
12. Choking					
13. Having to go to the hospital					
14. People in white uniforms					
15. Having somebody look at you					

Figure 9-1 Dental fear items from modified Children's Fear Survey Schedule. Reprinted by permission of Dr. Barbara Melamed.

parent can tell you, for example, how well the child typically copes with visits to the pediatrician. If the child usually resorts to tears and struggles and dreads every visit, this suggests limitations in coping skills which will also be apparent in the dental operatory. With children who have had prior dental experience, the parent can describe how well the child managed his behavior and emotions during the visit.

Don't overlook the child himself as a source of information about his own ability to cope. Dr. Barbara Melamed, a well-known psychologist who has studied children's behavior in the dental operatory, has developed a questionnaire which can be administered to the child before he enters the operatory.[17] The questionnaire consists of 15 items (Figure 9-1). For each question, the child uses a "fear thermometer" (Figure 9-2) to indicate how fearful he is. The child is given the following instructions:

> I would like you to tell me how afraid you are of some things. This is a fear thermometer. The bottom, Number 1, tells me you are not afraid at all. Number 2 tells me you are a little afraid. Number 3 tells me that you are a fair amount afraid. Number 4 tells me that you are pretty much afraid and Number 5 tells me that you are very afraid. For each thing I say, point to the number that tells me how afraid you are.

The questionnaire is scored by summing the child's score on all 15 items. Scores can range from 15 to 75. Dr. Melamed administered the questionnaire to a large group of children ages 5 to 13 and found that although scores varied with age and sex, the average score was 29—that is, an average score of about 2 on each item. If a child scores a 4 or 5 on

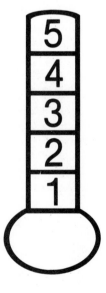

Figure 9-2 Fear Thermometer. Reprinted by permission of Dr. Barbara Melamed.

several items, thereby earning a score well above this average, you can be fairly sure that the child anticipates that he will have some difficulty coping with the demands of dental treatment.

Environments That Foster Coping

The physical environment is not simply a passive background for human behavior. The way in which space, furniture, and equipment are arranged can actively influence the emotions and behavior of people who enter the setting.

The dental environment—a busy place filled with new people, unusual objects, and strange noises—can be overwhelming to a young child. If the child is confronted with too much stimulation and, at the same time, must control his behavior in the reception area during a lengthy wait, he is likely to exhaust his coping ability even before he enters the operatory. For this reason, some thought should be given to providing for children's needs in the reception area. It is very difficult for small children to sit quietly for more than a few minutes, especially in adult-size chairs. A children's corner, with smaller furniture, bean-bag chairs, or cushions on the floor, will add to the comfort of your young patients. This also has the advantage of removing children from the immediate vicinity of other adult patients, not all of whom are fascinated by games of peek-a-boo or conversations that center around Pooh Bear.

Playthings for the children's area should be selected carefully. Collections of small objects such as dollhouse furniture, puzzles, and blocks are attractive to children. Be warned, however, that while small toys are nicely suited to small hands, they also pose big housekeeping problems. In addition, it is difficult for a young child to understand that all toys must remain behind when he leaves, and tantrums sometimes follow this realization. Avoid toys that invite noise and physical activity. Large toy cars and trucks practically compel young children to propel them across the length and breadth of the reception area, despite repeated instructions to "play quietly."

A large blackboard, hung at child height, is appealing to most preschool and early-elementary-school children and is ideal for encouraging quiet play. Other suitable toys are books, self-contained games for a single player, and "Etch-a-Sketch" devices.

In the operatory itself, the trend toward streamlining the work area, placing most instruments and equipment out of sight, has made the operatory a less threatening environment and thus one in which it is easier for the child to learn and practice coping. Many children express particular fear of the dental tools and instruments. In fact, research has shown that, in some cases, the sight of the equipment has an adverse effect on inexperienced children.[18] One interesting study investigated the effects of a clinical versus a nonclinical environment on children's anxiety: Results showed that children who were treated in a "streamlined" operatory were less anxious than were children who were treated in an operatory in which tools and equipment were in full view.[19] Children were also less anxious if their first contact with dental staff took place in a nonclinical area rather than in the operatory.

In summary, the fewer strange and potentially threatening sights and sounds with which the child must cope, the greater the likelihood that he will successfully master the demands of the situation. Attention to environmental details can pay dividends in terms of the behavior and attitudes of child patients.

Helping Children Cope with Dental Treatment

If you were to spend an afternoon browsing through an assortment of journals aimed at dental professionals, you would probably come across several articles suggesting different strategies for reducing children's fearful, uncooperative behavior during dental treatment—so many different strategies, in fact, that you might find yourself more confused than enlightened. The situation is made doubly confusing by the fact that many articles describe new methods, but few provide evidence that the methods actually work. Without this information, the task of choosing the most effective methods can be very difficult.

We can begin to bring order to this seeming chaos by asking the question, "What are the conditions that facilitate successful adjustment to new or stressful situations?" Briefly, coping is enhanced when a person: (a) knows what to expect; (b) knows exactly what will be expected of him; (c) has available some specific strategies for coping with stressful events; and (d) can practice coping and receive feedback.

From this analysis, it is apparent that to help the child learn to cope with dental treatment, we must

Prepare the child for what to expect

Explain what will be expected of the child

Teach the child to use specific coping skills

Provide feedback and reinforce coping behavior

Preparation for dental treatment.   The number and variety of preparatory approaches described in the professional literature suggests that dental professionals are well aware of the importance of preparing the child for the dental experience. One of the most widely used of these approaches is to send a letter to parents prior to the child's first visit, together with a card or a note sent to the child himself.

A useful preparatory letter to parents contains a brief description of what will happen at the first few visits (oral examination, prophylaxis, treatment planning, and so on). If it is office policy to allow parents into the operatory, guidelines to enable parents to participate as "silent partners" should be included. Tips for preparing the child should also be included. For example, parents should be encouraged to describe the dental staff as people who will help keep the child's teeth pretty, clean, and healthy, and who will help him learn to take good care of his teeth. Parents should be advised to avoid describing the dentist as "someone who pulls teeth." Because some parents have been known to threaten children with a trip to the dentist as punishment for misbehavior, it is a good idea to caution parents against this practice. The practice of sending a preparatory letter results in fewer broken appointments,[20] child behavior at the first visit tends to be more cooperative, and parents themselves view the letter as helpful.[21] This simple measure, therefore, appears to merit the minimal expense and effort involved.

On the other hand, a special "get-acquainted" visit solely for the purpose of familiarizing the child with the dental environment does *not* appear to yield appreciable benefits.[22] Because this method involves considerable time and effort, we do not recommend it.

When the child arrives for the first appointment, it is important to spend a few minutes with him in a nonclinic area like an office or conference room. A period of 10 to 15 minutes spent in friendly interaction with the child has been shown to produce considerable improvement in operatory entrance behavior.[23] In addition, you can use this time to observe the presence or absence of a variety of age-appropriate skills and behaviors and to obtain the child's responses to the Children's Dental Fear Survey.

The next step is to familiarize the young patient with exactly what will happen in the operatory. The popular Tell-Show-Do method is perhaps the best-known approach to providing information and exposure. As it is usually employed, this method consists of explaining each procedure, then demonstrating it on the professional or on an inanimate object. Simple language is used for the explanation and demonstration.*

A few researchers have reported modest improvements in the behavior of inexperienced children prepared for dental treatment with explanation-exposure approaches like Tell-Show-Do. If, however, this is the only preparatory method used, results are likely to be less than satisfactory with at least some children. There is even reason to believe

---

*Some professionals prefer to use a special vocabulary with children, substituting words like *electric pencil* for *handpiece*, *sleepy water* for *anesthesia*, and *rubber raincoat* for *rubber dam*.

that approaches that focus on fearful procedures and equipment can actually lead to *increases* in anxiety and uncooperative behavior in some dentally inexperienced children.[23,24] One investigator suggests that, "Too much information . . . [can lead] to heightened anxiety, perhaps caused by increasing the child's awareness of just how much may be done in a dental clinic."[25]

One way to prevent this problem and, at the same time, to provide the child with information and exposure is to allow fearful or inexperienced children to observe other children undergoing dental treatment and surviving the experience. Many clinicians routinely make use of such modeling procedures, and a substantial body of research evidence supports the effectiveness of this approach. An additional advantage of this method has come to light: If a mildly uncooperative child is used as a model, his own behavior improves when another child is present as an observer.[26] So although common sense would seem to dictate that only very calm, cooperative children should be used as models, good results can often be obtained with models whose behavior is a bit less than ideal.

Clinicians can take advantage of this "double-barrel" effect by scheduling appointments so that child patients have the opportunity to both observe and be observed by other children. If such scheduling is not possible, films or videotapes of children undergoing dental treatment are a useful substitute; research indicates that filmed models are about as effective as live models.

Teaching coping skills. When a child observes another child who is successfully coping in the dental operatory, he can see only the end product of that coping: calm and cooperative behavior. From observation alone, he cannot determine what coping strategies the child uses to remain calm during treatment. It is a wise precaution, therefore, to teach children what they can do to cope with the stress of dental treatment.

Many adult patients report that they cope with the stress and discomfort of dental treatment by meditating or using a variety of relaxation techniques. Others find that imagining themselves in a peaceful setting or thinking about pleasant events helps them maintain their composure. Patients who use such strategies rate dental treatment as less stressful than do those who do not.

Some clinicians and researchers have obtained good results through teaching children to relax by first stretching and tensing their muscles, then relaxing them.[27,28] Instructing children in deep breathing and encouraging them to imagine themselves in serene settings has also been described as helpful. But children are action oriented, so many do not respond as well as adults do to suggestions for relaxation or peaceful imagery. Better results are often obtained when children are encouraged to imagine themselves actively engaged in a favorite activity—the more strenuous and exciting, the better.

In one study illustrating the successful use of this approach, very fearful children were helped to overcome their fear of dental treatment by imagining themselves playing with their leaping, barking dogs.[29] They were told that they could keep their eyes closed during dental treatment (thereby aiding visualization while, at the same time, avoiding the sight of the frightening instruments). The children spent some time practicing and were praised for describing their visualizations. Then, with the dentist continuing to encourage active visualization, dental procedures were undertaken and accomplished easily and comfortably.

Children can also be encouraged to imagine themselves having an exciting adventure with their favorite television character or to imagine themselves watching their favorite television programs during dental treatment. This method is often used by practitioners of clinical hypnosis, with good results. Again, some practice should be given and the dental staff should provide praise and encouragement as the child describes what he is "seeing" or "doing."

Interestingly, allowing children to watch an actual television program during dental treatment does not seem to reduce fearful, uncooperative behavior. In one study, when children were simply permitted to watch videotaped cartoons displayed on an overhead monitor during treatment, there were no reductions in dental fear or uncooperative behavior.[3] Very different results ensued, however, when television viewing was made *contingent* on child behavior; that is, television viewing was permitted only when the child was calm and cooperative. If disruptive behavior such as crying or struggling occurred, television viewing was immediately interrupted by means of a switch on an extension cord. Television was made available again only when the child ceased the disruptive behavior. Children exposed to this simple method showed reductions of almost 50 percent in disruptive behavior, in comparison to their behavior at an initial baseline visit during which television was not available. These children also tended to report less fear of dental treatment after the visit, while children who were permitted to watch cartoons regardless of their behavior remained unchanged.

The results of a second study, which evaluated the effects of audiotaped stories as a means of helping children cope with dental treatment, provide even stronger support for the use of a contingent approach.[30] This study, like the preceding one, involved observing and recording the behavior of children undergoing dental treatment at an initial visit. At the second visit, children in both story-tape groups selected a tape from a small library of prerecorded tapes which included the adventures of Batman, Porky Pig, Star Trek, and the like. During dental treatment, children listened to the tapes through headphones. As in the first study, children in the contingent group were permitted to listen to the taped story only as long as they remained cooperative and quiet. If disruptive behavior occurred, the tape was interrupted. The results were clear and dramatic: The behavior of control-group children, who were not permitted to listen to tapes at all, actually worsened during the second visit. Children who were permitted to listen to tapes regardless of their behavior showed no change in behavior from the first to the second visit. In contrast, children in the contingent story-tape group showed reductions in disruptive behavior of 80 percent at the second visit. A change of this magnitude is both statistically and clinically meaningful and indicates clearly that this simple method is quite effective in helping children cope with dental treatment.

These findings are important not only because they demonstrate the usefulness of this easy, inexpensive method, but also because they suggest that simply distracting the child patient during dental treatment is *not* an effective way to promote cooperative behavior in the operatory. Others have also drawn this conclusion. In fact, studies have shown that the popular practice of talking about nondental matters in order to distract children during stressful or uncomfortable procedures actually leads to *increases* in fear-related behavior.[2]

Why should distraction prove useful with adults undergoing dental treatment (see Chapter 6), but not with children? The answer lies in the fact that the goals of intervention are different with child and adult patients. Since fearful adult patients do not usually scream, cry, and struggle to escape during treatment, we need not focus on helping them improve their overt behavior. Instead, our goal is to help them alter and control their thoughts and emotions when faced with the stress of dental treatment. Children, however, often "act out" their thoughts and emotions in their behavior, so, with this group, we are faced with the task of producing improvements not only in emotions and thoughts, but also in overt behavior.

There is no reason to believe that distraction techniques are useful tools for shaping new behaviors. Rather, as discussed in Chapter 8, an enormous body of evidence indicates that behavior change is facilitated by the prompt delivery of feedback and consequences. The use of feedback and reinforcement in the operatory will be discussed in a subsequent section.

Parents as a source of support.   Should the parent be present while you are teaching a child patient how to cope with dental treatment? Among those who have studied ways to help children cope with medical and dental procedures, some have convincingly urged that parents be actively involved as participants, especially with young children. To go a step further, it even seems desirable to offer parents the opportunity to remain in the operatory with their children during dental treatment. Because parents are the young child's primary source of emotional support, it is logical to assume that the reassuring presence of a parent should help the child cope in an unfamiliar and unsettling situation.

Several lines of research provide solid support for this assumption. For example, over 20 years ago, Dr. Spencer Frankl, a dentist at Tufts University, studied the behavior of 112 young children with and without mothers present.[4] Dr. Frankl found that children's reactions to dental treatment were more favorable when the mother was present in the operatory. This was particularly true of young children (under 5 years of age). At the University of Connecticut, a dentist-researcher Larry Venham has also explored this question, but from a slightly different angle.[31] In his investigation, Dr. Venham gave parents and children the option to remain together and found that the majority of parent-child pairs preferred to remain together, at least during the first few visits.

Why, then, do the majority of dentists prefer to exclude parents from the operatory? Many argue that the parent's presence is disruptive and interferes with rapport between dentist and child. No doubt some of these dentists have heard about or actually experienced difficulties with anxious or punitive parents whose presence seemed to increase the child's anxiety and disruptive behavior.

It is certainly true that not every parent can offer emotional support to a child undergoing dental treatment—in fact, some parents strongly prefer to remain in the reception area when their child is treated. If parents are offered the choice of remaining outside or accompanying their child, however, and if those who choose to accompany the child into the operatory are provided with some simple ground rules for their behavior in the operatory, they can provide valuable support to a child who is learning to cope with the demands of dental treatment.

Feedback and reinforcement for coping.   The child's first attempts to cope with the dental setting and dental procedures are likely to be faltering and unsure. During this learning process, what the dental professional says and does can have a very marked effect on the outcome. Continued guidance and feedback are necessary if the child is to master the tasks of sitting still, remaining relaxed, holding his mouth open, and complying with directives.

Instructions to the child, an important component of guidance, should be clear and simple. Avoid rhetorical questions such as, "Would you like to open your mouth now?" Children often interpret rhetorical questions literally, as if answers were expected, so it is quite possible that the child, believing that he has a choice, will simply refuse. In fact, results of a particularly interesting and informative study conducted by researchers at the University of Washington indicated that this is exactly what is likely to happen.[2] The investigators found that child patients were more likely to respond with negative or fear-related behavior to rhetorical questions; straightforward directives, such as "Open your mouth," produced more positive behavior.

These researchers also found that specific feedback, which tells the child exactly what he has done well, results in less disruptive behavior than does general feedback. For example, the comment, "I like the way you hold your mouth open nice and wide," provides the child with more information than does the statement, "You're such a good patient."

When you praise a child for appropriate coping behavior, your nonverbal cues can be as important as what you say. Gentle physical contact seems to have a comforting effect on young children. It is disheartening to note that the University of Washington studies revealed that patting and stroking are relatively infrequent dentist behaviors with young children, because patting and stroking, even in the absence of words, tend to promote calm, cooperative behavior.[2,32] A smile and a gentle pat accompanying praise for appropriate behavior will enhance the effects of the verbal praise.

What can be said about the use of negative feedback or criticism in the dental operatory? Negative feedback for inappropriate behavior is really a form of punishment, and the results are not always predictable. As we shall discuss in the next section, punishment should be used with great caution in the dental setting.

The pitfalls of punishment. Positive consequences tend to strengthen behavior, while negative, or aversive, consequences following a behavior tend to weaken the behavior. If praise and encouragement following appropriate coping behavior lead to increases in cooperative behavior, will criticism or negative feedback following disruptive behavior lead to reductions in undesirable behavior? The relationship between behavior and negative or punishing consequences is not quite so straightforward. The results of at least two recent investigations have shown, for example, that criticizing, blaming, or belittling the child actually results in *increases* in fearful, uncooperative behavior.[2,33] Even as seemingly mild a behavior as telling a child what *not* to do is less effective in increasing cooperative behavior than telling the child what you *do* want him to do. Young children, especially, find it difficult to inhibit a behavior, and instructing them to do something is usually more effective than telling them to stop doing something.

Physically restraining a disruptive child is also an ineffective approach to helping children cope with dental treatment. Results of the University of Washington studies clearly indicated that fear-related behavior was most likely to occur when the child was restrained. This finding is of special importance to dental professionals because the use of restraint is endorsed by many pediatric dentists, at least under some circumstances. In one study, 86 percent of the pediatric dentists polled agreed that there are occasions when some degree of physical restraint is necessary.[34]

One method of physical restraint which appears to be accepted by many dentists is the so-called Hand-Over-Mouth (HOM) technique. This method, which is taught in the majority of postgraduate pedodontic training programs in this country, consists of restraining the disruptive child with a hand placed firmly over the child's mouth.[35] Some dentists—perhaps as many as 30 percent or more—also cover the child's nose so that the child cannot breathe. The child is told, "When you are quiet and still, I will take my hand away."

One writer has attempted to defend this technique by relabeling it in psychological terms as "flooding" or "response prevention."[35] The writer's use of both terms is incorrect, but in any case renaming the technique does not alter the fact that it is a punishment procedure and a particularly frightening one, especially if the airways are blocked. Severely punishing a child for his inability to cope with a threatening situation is not likely to teach him more effective coping strategies. Rather, as considerable research attests, it is likely to lead to heightened emotional arousal and may convince the child that the dental situation is one to be feared and avoided in the future.

Voice control is another child management technique that is taught in many, if not most, dental schools. This approach involves speaking in a loud, sharp voice to the uncooperative child patient. Again, the results of empirical investigation do not support a negative or punishment-oriented approach to child behavior during dental treatment. Attempting to coerce the child, threatening him, or acting in a gruff manner are usually completely ineffectual interventions; more importantly, though, these dentist behaviors are often followed by substantial increases in disruptive child behavior.[2] Weinstein noted that

> Dentists seem to use these procedures when they feel frustrated by the child. Often the dentist's voice indicates his or her frustration, which may further exacerbate the situation. Emotional reactions are usually reciprocal: the child's fear-related behavior causes the dentist's frustration, which in turn causes further fear-related behavior in the child.[2]

In summary, punishment procedures are generally ineffective in helping children learn to cope with dental treatment. These procedures can even lead to increases in fearful, disruptive behavior. Further, there is reason for concern about the effects of punitive methods on the child's future attitudes toward dentistry. Before you consider using aversive methods with a child patient, remember that many fearful, avoidant adult patients give a history of rough or traumatic dental experiences during childhood. Is it worth the risk?

REFERENCES

1. Ingersoll, B.D., Ingersoll, T.G., McCutcheon, W.R., and Seime, R.J. Behavioral dimensions of dental practice: A national survey. Unpublished manuscript, West Virginia University School of Dentistry, 1979.

2. Weinstein, P., Getz, T., Ratener, P., and Domoto, P. The effect of dentists' behaviors on fear-related behaviors in children. *Journal of the American Dental Association* 104: 32, 1982.

3. Ingersoll, B.D., Nash, D.A., Blount, R.L., and Gamber, C. Distraction and contingent reinforcement with pediatric dental patients. *Journal of Dentistry for Children* 51:203, 1984.

4. Frankl, S.M., Shiere, F.R., and Fogels, H.R. Should the parent remain with the child in the dental operatory? *Journal of Dentistry for Children* 29:150, 1962.

5. Wright, F.A., Lucas, J.O., and McMurray, N.E. Dental anxiety in five-to-nine-year-old children. *Journal of Pedodontics* 4:99, 1980.

6. Morgan, P.H., Wright, L.E., Ingersoll, B.D., and Seime, R.J. Children's perceptions of the dental experience. *Journal of Dentistry for Children* 47:243, 1980.

7. Shaw, O. Dental anxiety in children. *British Dental Journal* 139:134, 1975.

8. Bailey, P.M., Talbot, A., and Taylor, P.P. A comparison of maternal anxiety levels with anxiety levels manifested in the child dental patient. *Journal of Dentistry for Children* 40:277, 1973.

9. Johnson, R., and Baldwin, D.C. Relationship of maternal anxiety to the behavior of young children undergoing dental extraction. *Journal of Dental Research* 47:801, 1968.

10. Wright, G.Z., and Alpern, G.D. Variables influencing children's cooperative behavior at the first dental visit. *Journal of Dentistry for Children* 38:124, 1971.

11. Wright, G.Z., Alpern, G.D., and Leake, J.L. A cross-validation of variables affecting children's cooperative behavior. *Journal of the Canadian Dental Association* 39:268, 1973.

12. Gesell, A., and Ilg, F. *The child from five to ten.* New York: Harper and Brothers, 1946.

13. Piaget, J., and Inhelder, B. *The psychology of the child.* New York: Basic Books, 1969.

14. Thomas, A., and Chess, S. *Temperament and development.* New York: Brunner/Mazel, 1977.

15. Zabin, M., and Melamed, B.G. The relationship between parental discipline and children's ability to cope with stress. Cited in B.G. Melamed and L.J. Siegel, *Behavioral medicine: Practical applications in health care*, p. 338. New York: Springer Publishing Co., 1980.

16. Venham, L.L., Murray, P., and Gaulin-Kremer, E. Child-rearing variables affecting the preschool child's response to dental stress. *Journal of Dental Research* 58:2042, 1979.

17. Cuthbert, M.I., and Melamed, B.G. A screening device: Children at risk for dental fears and management problems. *Journal of Dentistry for Children* 49:432, 1982.

18. Melamed, B.G. Behavioral approaches to fear in dental settings. In *Progress in behavior modification*, Volume 7. Edited by M. Hersen, R.M. Eisler, and P.M. Miller. New York: Academic Press, 1979.

19. Swallow, J., Jones, J., and Morgan, M. The effects of environment on a child's reaction to dentistry. *Journal of Dentistry for Children* 42:43, 1975.

20. Hawley, B.P., McCorkle, A.D., Wittemann, J.K., and Van Ostenberg, P. The first dental visit for children from low socioeconomic families. *Journal of Dentistry for Children* 41:376, 1974.

21. Wright, G.Z., Alpern, G.D., and Leake, J.L. The modifiability of maternal anxiety as it relates to children's cooperative dental behavior. *Journal of Dentistry for Children* 40:265, 1973.

22. Pinkham, J.R., and Fields, H.W. The effects of preappointment procedures on maternal manifest anxiety. *Journal of Dentistry for Children* 43:180, 1976.

23. Sawtell, R.O., Simon, J.F., and Simeonsson, R.J. Effects of five preparatory methods upon child behavior during the dental visit. *Journal of Dentistry for Children* 41:37, 1974.

24. Melamed, B.G., Yurcheson, R., Fleece, L., Hutcherson, S., and Hawes, R. Effects of film modeling on the reduction of anxiety-related behaviors in individuals varying in level of previous experience in the stress situation. *Journal of Consulting and Clinical Psychology* 46:1357, 1978.

25. Herbertt, R., and Innes, J. Familiarization and preparatory information in the reduction of anxiety in child dental patients. *Journal of Dentistry for Children* 46:319, 1979.

26. Williams, J., Hurst, M., and Stokes, T. Decreasing uncooperative behavior in young dental patients through the observation of and by peers. Paper presented at the annual meeting of the American Psychological Association, Los Angeles, California, 1981.

27. Siegel, L.J., and Peterson, L. Stress reduction in young dental patients through coping skills and sensory information. *Journal of Consulting and Clinical Psychology* 48:785, 1980.

28. Peterson, L., and Shigetomi, C. The use of coping techniques to minimize anxiety in hospitalized children. *Behavior Therapy* 12:1, 1981.

29. Ayer, W.A. Use of visual imagery in needle phobic children. *Journal of Dentistry for Children* 40:41, 1973.

30. Ingersoll, B.D., Nash, D.A., and Gamber, C. The use of contingent audiotaped material with pediatric patients. *Journal of the American Dental Association* 109:717, 1984.

31. Venham, L.L., Bengston, D., and Cipes, M. Parent's presence and the child's response to dental stress. *Journal of Dentistry for Children* 45:37, 1978.

32. Weinstein, P., Getz, T., Ratener, P., and Domoto, P. Dentists' responses to fear- and nonfear-related behaviors in children. *Journal of the American Dental Association* 104:38, 1982.

33. Melamed, B.G., Bennett, C.G., Jerrell, G., Ross, S.L., Bush, J.P., Hill, C., Courts, F., and Ronk, S. Dentists' behavior management as it affects compliance and fear in pediatric patients. *Journal of the American Dental Association* 106:324, 1983.

34. The Association of Pedodontic Diplomates. Technique for behavior management—A survey. *Journal of Dentistry for Children* 39:368, 1972.

35. Davis, M.J., and Rombom, H.M. Survey of the utilization of and rationale for Hand-Over-Mouth (HOM) and restraint in postdoctoral pedodontic education. *Pediatric Dentistry* 1:87, 1979.

10

The Elderly Patient

Michael J. Geboy

Today's health professionals will find that the elderly make up an ever-increasing percentage of their patients. Unfortunately, there are many stereotypes about this time of life, perhaps more than for any other. As a health professional, you must be able to separate the myths from the realities of later life. Our purpose in this chapter is to provide you with the information you need in order to treat your elderly patients most effectively.

WHO ARE THE ELDERLY?

Old age is usually defined in chronological terms. In our society, because of social security and medicare, the sixty-fifth birthday has assumed special significance as a milestone heralding entry into "old age." When individuals reach this landmark age, they become members of a new social group. They are afforded certain social privileges, such as health care benefits and discounts on medications and other purchases, but they must also live with new restrictions on their behavior. While chronological age is a useful way of defining old age for social purposes, it is much less useful for helping us understand other aspects of functioning, such as general health, physical status, and mental functioning. As we shall discuss, the process of normal aging involves many biological and psychological changes. Although these changes will eventually take place in all of us, there are significant individual differences in the rate at which they occur. Declines in bodily functioning may begin relatively early for some individuals but may not take place until much later for others. Consequently, two 65-year-olds, while members of the same age group, might be functionally quite different from each other. For example, although speed of response generally declines with age, some older adults are actually able to perform more rapidly than are many younger people.

Thus, the point at which a person enters old age is difficult to isolate. For a variety of social purposes, our culture has fixed this point at the individual's sixty-fifth birthday. As an indicator of a person's physical or psychological status, however, chronological age must not be relied upon too heavily.[1]

THE ELDERLY IN SOCIETY

Our society, like that of most Western nations, is aging. In 1980, some 25 million persons were aged 65 and older, accounting for approximately 11 percent of the total population. In comparison, the elderly made up only 4 percent of the population at the turn of the century. Population experts predict that the current trend is likely to continue into the future: It is projected that by 1990 there will be approximately 30 million people aged 65 and older; they will make up approximately 12 percent of the population. Moderate growth of this age group is expected to continue until about the end of the first decade of the twenty-first century, when the number of older adults will soar as the "baby boom generation" reaches retirement age.[2]

What are the reasons for this change in the age structure of our population? One factor is the declining birth rate in the United States. During the 1950s, for example, our population grew by about 18.5 percent. By the 1970s the rate of growth had slowed to about 11 percent, and during the present decade the growth rate is expected to be only about 10 percent.

The second major factor accounting for the current change in age structure is increased longevity. During the past 100 years, life expectancy—that is, the average number of years that people born in a given year can expect to live—has increased tremendously, both in the United States and in other Western nations. At the beginning of this century, the average life expectancy in the United States was about 49 years. By 1974, it had risen to 76 years for women and 68 years for men.[3]

Contrary to a popular myth, only about 5 percent of the elderly reside in institutions at any one point in time,[1] and most of the institutionalized elderly are aged 75 years and older. The majority of older people live in independent households. The majority of men aged 65 and older are married and live with their wives. Only about one out of seven is widowed. In contrast, over one-half of elderly women are widowed and about one-third live alone.[4]

With retirement, income and standard of living usually decline. While not all of the elderly are poor, they are, as a group, generally worse off than the rest of the population; nearly 75 percent are at the poverty level.[1] In general, elderly blacks have lower incomes than elderly whites, and a larger proportion of elderly blacks are at the poverty level. Similarly, elderly women have lower incomes than elderly men.

SENSORY AND PERCEPTUAL CHANGES IN OLD AGE

We interact with other individuals and with the environment through our senses. The senses are our "windows to the world," and sensory deficits can leave us isolated and alone. For this reason, there has been considerable interest in how our sensory capacities change with age. Because of their significance, much research has focused on understanding age-related changes in vision and hearing. In contrast, relatively little can be said with certainty about the effects of aging on our other senses.

Vision

With advancing age, the incidence of visual problems increases. Visual acuity (the sharpness of vision) shows relatively little change up until the age of 40 or 50, but there is a general decline after this age. By the age of 70, poor vision, if it is not corrected, is the rule rather than the exception.[5]

Many elderly persons experience a loss in the ability to focus on nearby objects, a condition termed *presbyopia* (far-sightedness). In general, the near point (the closest distance at which an object can be viewed without blur) becomes further away as we get older. This is, for the most part, the result of two changes in the eye. First, there is a decline in the elasticity of the lens of the eye; second, the eyeball itself changes shape. Both of these structural changes result in the projection of a blurred image onto the retina.

There is also some evidence that the speed of accommodation (the ability to focus on objects at different distances) decreases with age. In tests in which subjects first focus on a nearby object and then shift focus to a distant object, the time interval required to have the distant object in focus increases in older adults.[6]

Older people generally require greater levels of illumination than do younger people. In order to see well, sufficient light must reach the retina; with advancing age, a number of changes occur in the eye that reduce the amount of light admitted. The pupil of the eye is smaller in the older adult, so less light is admitted. In addition, the lens of the eye yellows, reducing the amount of light transmitted to the retina. Finally, the vitreous humor, the fluid-like substance filling the eyeball, becomes more opaque with age. Together, these changes result in a significant increase in the amount of light elderly people need in order to see clearly.

A related area of visual performance is dark adaptation. Studies have shown that older adults see less well in the dark and take longer to adjust to it.[7] Older adults also appear to be more susceptible to the effects of glare. Studies have shown that sensitivity to glare is slight up until about the age of 40, but it increases significantly between ages 40 and 70.

Change in color perception is another noticeable effect of aging. In particular, older adults have greater difficulty perceiving and discriminating among the shorter wavelengths of light—that is, the blues, greens, and violet. Colors at the other end of the spectrum—the reds and yellows—tend to be less affected. Although there may be other reasons, the primary cause of this distortion in color perception appears to be the yellowing of the lens of the eye. The lens acts somewhat like a filter on a camera lens so that shorter wavelengths are absorbed while the longer wavelengths are transmitted to the retina.

These changes in visual functioning have considerable practical significance. Reduced color sensitivity may make it difficult for the patient to deal with color-coded objects, while decreased acuity and farsightedness may make it more difficult for the patient to read instructions and medication labels. Reduced dark adaptation and increased sensitivity to glare make night driving difficult, so many older people restrict their driving after dark. Thus, it is helpful to schedule dental appointments so that the patient can get home before dark.

Audition

The changes in hearing that occur with advancing age are of perhaps greater practical significance than are the visual changes. The incidence of hearing loss increases with age, although, as is the case with visual impairments, there are significant individual differences. Approximately 30 percent of the older adult population show some sign of hearing loss.[8] Recent studies indicate that approximately 13 percent of those aged 65 and older show advanced signs of *presbycusis*, a progressive loss of hearing for higher frequency tones that occurs as a result of nerve degeneration. The ability to detect small changes in pitch also tends to decline with advancing age.

As might be expected, these changes in auditory perception affect the older individual's ability to discriminate speech, particularly when there are distortions or competing noises, such as the sound of the dental drill. Because of the major role hearing plays in communication, social interaction, and a host of everyday activities, auditory impairment can have a negative impact on the older person's adaptive and social functioning. Hearing-impaired individuals are unaware of many environmental warning signals. In addition, hearing deficits can undermine the ability to maintain normal interpersonal relations.[9] Self-consciousness and embarrassment over the deficit can cause the elderly individual to avoid social situations, leading to increased isolation and loneliness. Emotional disturbance, particularly depression, has been found to be related to chronic hearing loss,[10] and paranoid tendencies may become accentuated by a hearing problem, resulting in increased suspiciousness and hostility. In terms of personal adjustment, an interview study of nearly 300 centenarians revealed that it is more difficult to adjust to hearing loss than to loss of sight.[11] A mild-to-moderate hearing loss is often not readily apparent to others; thus, a failure to respond or a tendency to respond inappropriately during conversation is apt to be misconstrued as antisocial behavior or even as senility rather than simply as the result of a hearing problem. Later in this chapter, we will discuss some of the things you can do to help improve communication with the hearing-impaired elderly.

Taste, Smell, and Other Senses

Compared with vision and hearing, relatively little can be said with certainty about the effects of aging on the senses of taste and smell. There is some evidence to suggest that taste sensitivity remains relatively constant until the later 50s and then declines.[12] Recent studies suggest that olfactory sensitivity shows little, if any, decrement in later adulthood, at least for healthy individuals.[13,14]

To the extent that taste sensitivity does decline in later adulthood, the loss can have important implications. Eating becomes less pleasurable, because the loss of sensitivity can result in foods tasting bland. In addition, dietary restrictions necessitated by chronic health problems, such as the low-salt diets of patients with hypertension, might restrict the use of substances that enhance the taste of food.

There is currently little clear-cut evidence that aging affects other senses, such as touch and sensitivity to pain. The vestibular senses, on the other hand, do appear to decline in function. Dizziness is more frequent among elderly people and is one of the major causes of injury in this population.[15]

PSYCHOLOGICAL CHANGES IN THE ELDERLY

Learning and Memory

The research on learning and memory in later adulthood is complex and often difficult to interpret. There is substantial evidence, however, that elderly people do not perform as well as young persons do on either learning or memory tasks.[16] Nevertheless, it is important to keep these findings in perspective. The vast majority of older people are able to adapt reasonably well to their declining cognitive abilities. Unless the deficits are severe—such as the memory deficits that accompany organic brain damage—most people are able to continue handling their own affairs with relatively little difficulty throughout most of later life.[17]

Sexual Behavior

One of the most prevalent stereotypes regarding the later years is that sexual desire and sexual activity cease to exist. Related to this is the belief that sexual behavior should cease with entrance into later adulthood.[18]

How true are these stereotypes? Research has shown that the frequency of sexual thoughts does decline with advancing age. In one study, for example, individuals between the ages of 8 and 99 were asked to respond to the question, "What were you thinking about over the past 5 minutes?"[19] The questionnaire was completed by nearly 4500 people in a variety of settings. In general, the frequency of both focused and in-passing thoughts about sex was found to be significantly related to age. Thoughts about sex reached greatest frequency during adolescence, remained relatively stable during the early adult years, then gradually declined.

While there is a decline in the frequency of sexual thoughts, sexual interest and activity continue well into the later years. In one large-scale study of individuals between 60 and 94 years of age, about 80 percent of a group of healthy men reported continuing sexual interest, while 70 percent reported that they were still sexually active. Ten years later these same individuals were interviewed again, and little decline in interest was reported; however, the proportion who were sexually active had dropped to 25 percent.[18]

In a similar sample of healthy women, approximately one-third reported continuing sexual interest and about one-fifth were still regularly active at the time of the initial interviews. At the time of the second interview ten years later, the proportion interested in sex remained about the same, as did the percentage who were sexually active. Another interesting finding was that the likelihood of continued sexual expression in later adulthood was substantially greater for people who were highly interested and sexually active in their younger years. People who were very active in earlier adulthood tend to continue sexual behavior into their later years.

Mental Health and Aging

The stresses of the later years present severe adaptation difficulties for some elderly people. Life crises such as widowhood, sensory loss, and retirement affect all older adults to an extent and may be a factor in the development of a variety of functional disturbances. The elderly are also subject to organic disorders as a result of degenerative changes in the brain.

The incidence of psychiatric disorders generally increases with age. For instance, a study by the National Institute of Mental Health revealed that the number of new cases of psychopathology of all types ranged from 2.3 cases per 100,000 population in the under-15 group, to 93 cases per 100,000 in 35-to-54-year-olds, to 236.1 cases per 100,000 in those over age 65.[20] Other estimates suggest that approximately 15 percent of the elderly population of the United States suffer from some level of psychopathology.[21] The proportion of people who suffer from psychiatric disorders severe enough to require hospitalization also increases significantly with advancing age, due primarily to a greater incidence of disorders involving impaired brain functioning. Brain disorders account for an increasingly larger proportion of the total amount of mental illness with advancing age. In the 65-to-74-year-old group, for example, more than half of the individuals in mental hospitals are there because of problems not related to organic brain disorders. In the 75-and-older group, on the other hand, the organic brain disorders account for over half of the cases in psychiatric hospitals.[22]

Depressions are the most common of the functional psychiatric disorders in the elderly. Depressed individuals complain of a variety of psychological and physical symptoms. Psychological symptoms of depression include difficulty in making decisions, feelings of helplessness, and diminished self-esteem. Also prominent are inhibition of activity, and feelings of sadness and pessimism. Physical signs include loss of appetite, significant weight loss, early morning fatigue, sleeplessness, and constipation.

Although milder forms of depression can often be treated successfully with psychotherapy, drug therapy is frequently necessary in more severe cases. Antidepressant drugs can cause serious side effects in older people, however, and such factors as decreased metabolic rate in the elderly can prolong drug action or produce exaggerated effects.[23]

Suicide is also a problem among the aged. People over the age of

65 account for over 30 percent of all suicides.[21] The highest rate of suicide, according to recent studies, occurs among white males in their 80s. The thought of suicide should be taken seriously when it occurs in older persons, because elderly adults are much more successful than are younger people at actually committing suicide.[24] Unlike younger people, when aged individuals attempt suicide, they almost always intend to die.[25]

Why do the elderly commit suicide? There are several reasons.[20] Particularly among older white males, suicide may be, in part, the result of the severe loss of status and self-esteem that affects white males, who, as a group, held the greatest power and influence in society during their younger years. Suicide may also be used as a way of exerting some measure of control over death; while one cannot escape the certainty of death, one can influence when and how it will happen. Finally, suicide can be the result of a rational or philosophical decision; that is, an elderly person might commit suicide to avoid pain or physical helplessness and dependency, or to spare surviving family members the costs of a long-term illness.

Next to depression, paranoid reactions are the most common psychiatric disturbance in older adults. Paranoid reactions most frequently occur in older people who have various types of sensory losses, particularly in those with hearing losses. Hypochondrical reactions have also been found to increase in frequency with advancing age. A related but normal feature of later adulthood is an increase in "body monitoring."[23] Because the older individual's body no longer functions as efficiently or automatically as it did when he was young, he must pay more attention to bodily processes.

Organic brain syndromes represent the second major class of psychiatric disorders among the elderly. Unlike the functional disorders, for which no physical causes have been identified, organic brain syndromes are the result of trauma to the brain. The symptoms associated with organic brain disease are related to the degree of brain impairment. Among the major symptoms are disturbance and impairment of short- and long-term memory; impairment of intellectual functioning; impairment of judgment; and problems of orientation.[23]

Physicians have recently begun to distinguish between *reversible* (acute) and *irreversible* (chronic) brain syndromes. Estimates suggest that between 10 and 20 percent of organic brain syndromes in elderly patients are reversible. Reversible organic brain syndromes are thought to be due to a temporary, or reversible, malfunction of the brain, and a number of potential causes have been identified. Congestive heart failure, for example, can result in an undersupply of essential oxygen and other nutrients to the brain. Malnutrition, due to poor nutritional habits and the inability to chew food, might be involved. Many older adults take a variety of drugs for chronic illnesses, and drug reactions can result in brain cell malfunctions. Finally, diabetes and other metabolic disorders can be involved. A current problem in the field is the misdiagnosis of reversible organic brain syndromes as chronic disorders, with the result that older people are sometimes sent to long-term care institutions and written off as untreatable; with proper treatment, however, many can show partial or even complete recovery.

Dealing with Death

When we are young, we think in terms of how long we have lived. When we are old, we begin to think in terms of how long we have left to live. In later life, one is faced with the following three important tasks:

Dealing with the realization of death as an unavoidable event and with the prospect of one's own imminent death

Coping with the loss of spouse, friends, and other loved ones

Facing the dying process itself

There are many ways of dealing with the prospect of one's own imminent death. For some, death is not viewed with dismay: "Many persons have the ability to cross into old age and face death with a conscious, though perhaps unverbalized, feeling of satisfaction with past achievements and a sense of contentment with life as they have lived it."[26] Others, less able to contemplate their own deaths, use defense mechanisms, such as denial or withdrawal through alcohol or drugs, to avoid a clear awareness of death. For still others, a belief in life after death helps them to deal with the prospect of death. Planning for the disposition of one's material possessions is often a tangible indicator that one has accepted the fact of death, regardless of how near or distant it may be.

Psychologists have found that the relative nearness to death of the elderly often triggers a process termed the *life review*, which usually consists of increased reminiscence, self-reflection, nostalgia, and often mild regret over past wrongs.[27] In some instances, however, there may be extreme preoccupation with the past, and one may feel great guilt, depression, and despair over one's past life. On the other hand, the process of reviewing one's life can have positive consequences, such as acceptance of the ending of life, pride in accomplishment, and a sense of serenity. Through this process, the individual may become ready, but in no hurry, to die.

The loss of a spouse or other loved ones initiates the grief process. Grief reactions to the death of others can range from mild to very intense. The most common symptoms of grief include crying, depressed feelings, difficulty sleeping, poor concentration and memory, loss of appetite, and reliance on tranquilizers or sleeping pills.[28] More severe symptoms, such as hallucinations, anxiety attacks, and physical illness, are sometimes reported. Studies of bereaved persons suggest that they are more susceptible to physical illness and death. In addition to the grief process that follows the death of a loved one, there is also a phenomenon termed *anticipatory grief*, in which many of the grief symptoms are exhibited before the actual loss of a loved one. It has been suggested that anticipatory grief might be more common today than it once was because of a shift from relatively swift to more lingering deaths, such as those due to cancer and other chronic conditions, and because of medical advances that have made it possible to prolong life.[29]

What can be done to aid the grieving person? At least during the first month or so, assisting the bereaved person with immediate plans is often the most helpful thing one can do. The lonely hours of evening and night are often reported as worst for the bereaved to endure, so companionship during these hours can be especially supportive.[30]

HEALTH AND DISEASE

As we age, the pattern of illness changes. Certain types of disease decrease in frequency, while other types occur more frequently. The incidence of acute illness, for example, is highest during childhood and adolescence and tends to decline during the adult years. The incidence of chronic disease, on the other hand, increases as we age. Heart disease, for example, is the leading cause of death and limitation of activity in people aged 65 and older.[30] Hypertension also tends to increase with age, as does arthritis. Finally, older adults exhibit an increased susceptibility to infections. The fact that elderly people are more likely to suffer from multiple conditions complicates the health picture in later adulthood.

These changes in the pattern of illness have several implications for the dental professional. First, individuals with chronic disease are likely to be on long-term medication regimens and may be taking several different medications simultaneously. For this reason, it is important to take a thorough medical history so that any factors that might complicate dental treatment can be identified. Increased susceptibility to infection and limited range of activity as a result of chronic conditions such as arthritis are also factors that must be taken into account during treatment and when planning oral hygiene programs.

Patterns of Oral Disease

The National Center for Health Statistics has conducted surveys designed to provide information about the incidence of oral disease in the United States population.[31] According to their studies, the incidence of periodontal disease increases with age. For example, approximately 37 percent of dentulous adults between the ages of 45 and 64 exhibit advanced periodontal disease, compared with 50 percent of those between 65 and 74. Edentulism also increases with age. Approximately 46 percent of those aged 65 to 74 are edentulous, compared with about 75 percent of those aged 75 and older. Although edentulism will continue to be a common problem for the elderly, there is some indication that the incidence is declining. It now appears that life-long use of fluoride and better dental care will result in an increase in the number of people who retain their natural dentition throughout their lives.

Dryness of the mouth, while not a disease in itself, is a common complaint among the elderly.[31] Several factors appear to be responsible for this condition, including mouth breathing, thicker mucus, and decreased saliva production.

These changes in oral health have several important implications for the geriatric patient. Edentulism and dryness of the mouth influence both the quantity and type of food consumed, so significant changes in diet can result. Individuals who suffer from these conditions often select soft, self-lubricating foods, such as gelatin. Such foods are easier to eat, but they often lack essential nutrients. While dentures are an improvement, they are much less effective than natural dentition. To reach the same level of mastication, for instance, a denture wearer must chew food four times longer than a person with teeth would have to. These diet alterations can have a deleterious impact upon the elderly person's nutritional status. One recent study revealed that the diets of a group of edentulous patients were deficient in more than one-third of the nutrients analyzed; further, even when patients were given new dentures, their diets were still inadequate.[32]

Apart from its effects on physical health, edentulism is often accompanied by loss of self-esteem, due in part to changes in appearance. Fortunately, dentures can result in improvements in the elderly person's appearance and sense of well-being.

Beliefs about Aging and Health

Many people, including the elderly themselves, believe that disease always accompanies the aging process. Although the gradual physiological changes that occur with age increase the vulnerability to disease, many elderly maintain their health well into the later years. The development of many of the chronic diseases that affect the elderly, including dental disease, is strongly influenced by environmental factors and by personal habits and behaviors. Life-long exposure to environmental pollution, certain personal habits such as alcohol consumption and cigarette smoking, and the absence of preventive activities such as adequate oral hygiene, are all important factors in the development of chronic disease in the later years. Unfortunately, the expectancy of ill health in old age serves to lessen motivation to change one's habits. If the loss of teeth, for example, is thought to be normal, little effort will be expended to avoid it. Health professionals are in a unique position to lead the way toward the development of new attitudes that can significantly improve the level of health in the later years.

COMMUNICATING WITH THE AGED PATIENT

The older adult must communicate with others to fulfill both physical and social needs. Communication is a complex process at all stages of life, but some of the characteristics of aging can make it more difficult to communicate effectively. As a health professional, you must recognize and accommodate to these characteristics in order to ensure that your interchanges will be successful and satisfying.

Elderly adults may be subject to many speech and language impairments as a result of a variety of physiological changes and as a result of disease. For some individuals, problems in articulation can arise as a result of Parkinson's disease or cancer. Normal voice changes include decline in the frequency range and in vocal quality, particularly in the singing voice, and an increased frequency of vocal strain and fatigue. Finally, an elderly person might experience expressive or receptive aphasia as a result of a stroke—that is, difficulty in using or understanding language.

Sensory impairments can also influence the aged person's ability to communicate. As we have discussed, the visual and auditory systems begin to decline during the process of aging. Hearing difficulties can cause the elderly person to be uncertain about what has been said to him, which can cause him to withdraw from an interchange rather than risk responding inappropriately. If the older person refuses to accept the hearing loss and instead blames his failure on the other person's speech, additional problems arise.

You can take several steps to counteract these sensory losses and improve your ability to communicate with the aged patient. When speaking with someone who has a hearing loss, for instance, remember that simply increasing the volume of your speech does not make it more intelligible. You can improve communication, however, by speaking slowly and facing the person so that he can lip-read. Turn off equipment while you are speaking, because hearing loss is exacerbated by the interference of other sounds. Another point to remember: Never come up to a hearing-impaired person from behind and tap him on the shoulder to get his attention; this will needlessly startle him. Instead, walk around and approach him from the front so that you can be seen. It can also be useful to find out whether the person hears better in one ear than the other.

Many younger people report a feeling of discomfort at the thought of touching an elderly person. For some, the changes in physical appearance that accompany aging are disconcerting to them. Some elderly people appear frail. Nevertheless, a reassuring touch can often communicate interest and caring more effectively than any words you offer.

Researchers have recently found that younger adults tend to simplify their language when speaking to the elderly, much as one does when talking to young children. Explanations, for example, often involve simpler words and are less complex. Why is this so? Other research suggests that it is because the elderly are generally perceived as less competent, so the language and concepts used are simplified.[33] This research was intended only to describe how we communicate with elderly people, but there is a lesson to be learned from it. Although hearing impairments and other handicapping conditions that are associated with old age might make speech changes necessary, we should not automatically assume that this is the case with all elderly people. When a competent and healthy older person is addressed in language that is more appropriate for use with a child, the message is likely to be perceived as patronizing and demeaning, which can, obviously, negatively impact the provider–patient relationship.

You also communicate with your elderly patients through the physical environment you create. The office environment, through its design, can communicate caring and concern, or can convey just the opposite. A building with steep steps and no ramps, for example, might just as well bear a sign saying "Elderly keep out!" because it is likely to be difficult or even impossible for the aged patient to enter. Seating accommodations are also important; chairs with firm cushions and sturdy arms make the task of seating one's less-strong elderly body less trying. Bathroom facilities with side-bars are becoming increasingly common and can help to compensate for the physical limitations of some elderly people. These and other prosthetic design features can significantly improve the aged person's ability to function in the dental office environment. Moreover, they communicate a message of understanding and concern to the patient.

Finally, patience is a cardinal virtue when you interact with the elderly. It is often difficult for the young, vigorous person to adjust to the slower pace at which the elderly person is apt to walk, speak, and behave. You might have to make a special effort to give older people the time they need to communicate with you by refraining from interrupting them or finishing their sentences for them. You will also have to pay special attention to your nonverbal cues. Remember that no matter how patient your words and tone of voice, a tapping foot and other telltale nonverbal signals convey a very clear message of impatience, which is likely to be perceived and believed.

Perhaps it will help you feel greater empathy for your elderly patients if you pause from time to time to remember that this is a stage of life that you, too, will one day enter. As the comedian W.C. Fields observed, "Growing old isn't so bad—when you consider the alternative!"

REFERENCES

1. Butler, R.N., and Lewis, M.I. *Aging and mental health* (2nd ed.). St. Louis: C.V. Mosby, 1977.

2. American Dental Association *Interim report of the American Dental Association's special committee on the future of dentistry.* Chicago: American Dental Association, 1982.

3. *Sourcebook on Aging* (2nd ed.). Chicago: Marguis Academic Media, 1979.

4. Murphy, J., and Florio, C. Older Americans: Facts and potential. In *The new old: Struggling for dental aging.* Edited by R. Gross, B. Gross, and S. Seidman. Garden City, N.Y.: Anchor Books, 1978.

5. Botwinick, J. *Aging and behavior.* New York: Springer Publishing Co., 1973.

6. Fozard, J.L., Wolf, E., Bell, B., McFarland, R.A., and K.W. Schaie, editors. *Handbook of the psychology of aging.* New York: Van Nostrand Reinhold, 1977.

7. Domey, R.G., McFarland, R.A., and Chadwick, E. Dark adaptation as a function of age and time: II. A derivation. *Journal of Gerontology* 15:267, 1960.

8. Schwartz, A.N., and Peterson, J.A. *Introduction to Gerontology.* New York: Holt, Rinehart & Winston, 1979.

9. Corso, J.F. Auditory perception and communication. In *Handbook of the psychology of aging.* Edited by J.E. Birren and K.W. Schaie. New York: Van Nostrand Reinhold, 1977.

10. Knapp, P.H. Emotional aspects of hearing loss. *Psychosomatic Medicine* 10:203, 1948.

11. Beard, B.B. Sensory decline in very old age. *Gerontological Clinics* 11:149, 1969.

12. Cooper, R.M., Bilash, I., and Zubek, J.P. The effect of age on taste sensitivity. *Journal of Gerontology* 14:56, 1959.

13. Engen, T. Taste and smell. In *Handbook of the psychology of aging.* Edited by J.E. Birren and K.W. Schaie. New York: Van Nostrand Reinhold, 1977.

14. Rovee, C.K., Cohen, R.Y., and Shlapack, W. Life-span stability in olfactory sensitivity. *Developmental Psychology* 11:311, 1975.

15. Kalish, R.A. *Late adulthood: Perspectives on human development.* Monterey, Calif.: Brooks/Cole, 1975.

16. Ahrenberg, D., and Robertson-Tchabo, E.A. Learning and aging. In *Handbook of the psychology of aging.* Edited by J.E. Birren and K.W. Schaie. New York: Van Nostrand Reinhold, 1977.

17. Hulicka, I.M. Cognitive functioning in late adulthood. *Selected documents in psychology.* American Psychological Association, 1979.

18. Pfeiffer, E. Sexual behavior in old age. In *Behavior and adaptation in late life* (2nd ed.). Edited by E.W. Busse, and E. Pfeiffer. Boston: Little, Brown, 1977.

19. Cameron, P., and Biber, H. Sexual thought throughout the life-span. *The Gerontologist* 13:144, 1973.

20. Butler, R.N. *Why survive? Being old in America.* New York: Harper & Row, Pub., 1975.

21. Pfeiffer, E. Psychopathology and social pathology. In *Handbook of the psychology of aging.* Edited by J.E. Birren and K.W. Schaie. New York: Van Nostrand Reinhold, 1977.

22. Busse, E.W., and Pfeiffer, E. Functional psychiatric disorders in old age. In *Behavior and adaptation in late life* (2nd ed.). Edited by E.W. Busse and E. Pfeiffer. Boston: Little, Brown, 1977.

23. Kart, C.S., Metress, E.S., and Metress, J.F. *Aging and health: Biologic and social perspectives.* Reading, Mass.: Addison-Wesley, 1978.

24. Gardner, E., Bahn, A.K., and Mach, M. Suicide and psychiatric care in the aging. *Archives of General Psychiatry* 10:547, 1963.

25. Benson, R.A., and Brodie, D.C. Suicide by overdoses of medicines among the aged. *Journal of the American Geriatric Society* 23:304, 1975.

26. Jeffers, F.C., and Verwoerdt, A. How the old face death. In *Behavior and adaptation in late life* (2nd ed.). Edited by E.W. Busse and E. Pfeiffer. Boston: Little, Brown, 1977.

27. Butler, R.N. The life review: An interpretation of reminiscence in the aged. *Psychiatry* 26:65, 1963.

28. Clayton, P.J., Halikes, J.A., and Maurice, W.L. The bereavement of the widowed. *Diseases of the Nervous System* 32:579, 1971.

29. Kastenbaum, R., and Costa, P.T., Jr. Psychological perspectives on death. *Annual Review of Psychology* 28:225, 1977.

30. Kimmel, D.C. *Adulthood and aging.* New York: John Wiley, 1974.

31. Basic data on dental examination findings of persons 1–74 years, U.S., 1971–1974. Series 11, No. 214, DHEW Publication (PHS) 9-1662, May, 1979.

32. Baxter, J.C. Nutrition and the geriatric edentulous patient. *Special Care in Dentistry* 1:259, 1981.

33. Tamir, L.M. *Communication and the aging process.* Elmsford, N.Y.: Pergamon Press, 1979.

11

The Handicapped Patient

Sanford J. Fenton
and Christina B. DeBiase

The handicapped population in the United States has been estimated at over 27 million.[1] Included are the medically compromised victims of stroke, acquired cardiac disease, and cancer), the aged, the chronically disabled (for example, those with cerebral palsy, muscular dystrophy, polio, impaired vision, or impaired hearing), the neurologically impaired (including patients with seizure disorders, mental retardation, and autism), and those with congenital abnormalities (such as Down's syndrome, heart disease, and rubella).

It is only during the last decade that the dental profession has seriously addressed the dental needs of the handicapped patient. Several barriers had prohibited members of the dental health professions from successfully treating these patients. Such obstacles included the following:

Office inaccessibility

Insufficient factual information concerning the care and needs of the handicapped patient

Inadequate curricula in dental schools and professional training programs

Apathy of parents or legal guardians toward dental needs

Noninclusion of dental professionals in total health care planning teams

Poor acceptance of the philosophy of preventive dentistry in the home, school, or professional dental environment

Lack of a coordinated effort by members of health professions on a national, state, and local level

Inadequate funding[2,3]

Efforts at alleviating these impediments have met with significant success. In 1968, Title I, Part B of Public Law 88-164 established funds for the development of university-affiliated facilities (UAFs) to offer specialized training in the comprehensive care of the handicapped patient. A few years later, in 1973, the Rehabilitation Act was passed. According to Section 504 of this act, it is illegal and discriminatory for health care providers to deny services to anyone simply on the basis of a handicapping condition. Federal regulations regarding this act have precise suggestions for the construction of programs and facilities in institutions of dental education, private dental offices, and other treatment facilities.[4]

The Academy of Dentistry for the Handicapped is an organization of dental professionals who have accepted responsibility for providing comprehensive dental care to a maximum number of handicapped individuals. *Special Care in Dentistry*, a periodical published by the American Dental Association, has made information pertaining to the management of handicapped patients available to dental personnel. In 1973, 11 dental schools received funding totalling $4.7 million from the Robert Wood Johnson Foundation to design programs to train dental students in the dental management of the nonhospitalized special patient.[5] The success of this pilot program led to the establishment of specific curriculum development guidelines which can be utilized by other dental institutions. These guidelines are also applicable to dental hygiene and dental assisting education.

COMMON HANDICAPPING CONDITIONS

Although it is not within the scope of this chapter to present an exhaustive list of all handicapping conditions, it is important that you be familiar with several of the more common disorders encountered in the dental office and with the management techniques necessary to successfully treat these patients.

Mental Retardation

Mental retardation is one of the more frequently occurring handicaps. The incidence of mental retardation in the United States is 3 percent, or approximately 6.5 million affected persons.[6] It is interesting to note that an overwhelming majority of retarded people—over 85 percent—reside in local community settings rather than in state facilities and institutions. You can see the potential for dental care this group represents for the dental professional who has the empathy and clinical skills needed to deal with the dental problems of the mentally retarded.

Mentally retarded individuals are classified into the following four subgroups: mildly, moderately, severely, and profoundly retarded. Intelligence quotients (I.Q. scores) are not the sole criterion, but they are helpful in evaluating the severity of the retardation. A score of 100 on an I.Q. test represents an average level of intelligence. *Mildly retarded* individuals score between 52 and 67. As a group, the mildly retarded account for 85 percent of all retarded individuals. With proper education and habilitation, mildly retarded people can function at the third to sixth grade level. *Moderately retarded* individuals (those with I.Q. scores in the range between 36 and 51) represent 10 percent of all retarded people. They can achieve a first to second grade level of functioning with intensive training. The *severely retarded* (with I.Q. scores of 20 to 35) and the *profoundly retarded* (with I.Q. scores of less than 20) respond minimally to their environments and require supervision and care for their personal needs. Many of these individuals, especially those who function at a profoundly retarded level, require institutional care. The severely and profoundly retarded account for 5 percent of the retarded.[7]

The mentally retarded often have physiological problems in addition to deficits in intellectual functioning. The more severely retarded may exhibit bizarre behavior patterns, such as head banging, biting, and other self-stimulatory behaviors. The retarded often have short attention spans, sensory defects, poor social adjustment, and concurrent congenital anomalies. You must be aware of these potential problems in order to design an appropriate treatment protocol.

Cerebral Palsy

Cerebral palsy is an example of a physically disabling condition. Cerebral palsy is caused by a nonprogressive, permanent injury to the brain. The major clinical symptom is motor disturbance, but associated handicaps, such as mental retardation, sensory defects, and convulsions, are often seen. The incidence of cerebral palsy in the United States is 0.7 percent. It remains one of the leading causes of crippling in children.

The two most common types of cerebral palsy are *spasticity* and *athetosis*; together they account for over 75 percent of all cases. The spastic individual exhibits increased muscle tone, which causes an exaggerated contraction of the muscle when it is stretched. The patient suffering from athetosis exhibits slow, writhing movements of the extremities.[8]

Oral manifestations of cerebral palsy include increased periodontal disease, class II malocclusions, and a high incidence of oral habit disorders (including mouth breathing, tongue thrusting, and bruxism).

Seizure Disorders

Patients with seizure disorders, or epilepsy, are frequently encountered among the handicapped population. The incidence of epilepsy in the general population is 1 percent.

Classification depends on the clinical manifestations of the seizure episodes. *Grand mal seizures* are the most severe variant of this disorder. Grand mal seizure episodes are characterized by violent, generalized muscular spasms, loss of consciousness, and, sometimes, cyanosis. Individual seizure episodes rarely last longer than 5 to 10 minutes. Following a grand mal attack, patients may appear disoriented and depressed or suffer from headaches or nausea.

Petit mal seizures are characterized by transient lapses of consciousness. There may be concurrent minor motor dysfunctions, such as quivering of the eyelids, tremors of the extremities, and nodding of the head. Individual episodes rarely last longer than 30 seconds. Victims of petit mal seizures may experience up to several hundred seizure episodes daily. Other types of seizure disorders include focal, thalamic, and hypothalamic seizures.

Oral manifestations of this neurological disorder include fractured incisors and gingival hypoplasia. Fractured incisors often result from unintentional self-inflicted trauma to the craniofacial region following loss of balance during an acute attack. In addition, well-meaning but misdirected "good samaritans" sometimes cause injury to the oral cavity and dentition by trying to force apart the jaws after the onset of generalized convulsions.

Drug-induced hyperplasia is another common finding in the epileptic patient. Phenytoin sodium (Dilantin), a frequently used anticonvulsant medication, has been shown to cause hyperplasia of the gingiva, particularly in the absence of a good oral hygiene regimen. It is critical to stress the importance of good oral hygiene to your epileptic patients in an attempt to reduce the possibility or severity of Dilantin-induced gingival hyperplasia.

Oncology

The treatment of patients with blood dyscrasias can be challenging to the dental professional. This group encompasses, but is not limited to, individuals with leukemia, hemophilia, cyclic neutropenia, anemia, and thrombocytopenia. These disorders can lead to severe oral complications. These patients are more prone to infection, ulceration, delayed healing, and abnormal bleeding of the oral cavity. It is crucial to take a thorough medical history and to seek medical consultation before initiating dental treatment. The patients must be counseled on proper oral hygiene procedures to reduce the possibility of dental infections and spontaneous gingival bleeding. Prevention of dental disease, while important for the normal, healthy person, is paramount for the person with a serious blood dyscrasia.[9]

Sensory Disabilities

One of the most rewarding experiences for the dental professional who treats patients with special needs is the successful management of the patient with a severe visual or hearing impairment. The major obstacle to the successful management of the sensory-disabled patient is establishment of adequate communication (see Chapter 10). Of the two disabilities, deafness usually represents the greater challenge for the dental professional.

Numerous etiological factors are associated with deafness. Prenatal factors implicated in deafness include premature birth, Rh incompatability, maternal infections, congenital defects, and birth trauma. Postnatal factors include adverse reactions to medications, infections, trauma, and auditory nerve or auditory cortex damage. Heredity is also an etiological factor in deafness.

Deafness can be classified according to the location of the injury or defect. *Conductive* hearing loss refers to problems that involve the outer or middle ear, while *sensorineural* loss involves damage to the structures of the inner ear, auditory nerve, or auditory center of the brain.[10]

Blindness also has multiple etiologies. Prenatal factors include maternal infections, congenital abnormalities, and prematurity. Postnatal causes include trauma, diabetes mellitus, glaucoma, cataracts, retrolental fibroplasia, and leukemia.[10]

Cardiovascular Conditions

Cardiovascular patients include those patients with a history of rheumatic fever, rheumatic heart disease, congenital heart disease, atherosclerosis, hypertension, and congestive heart failure.

Taking a thorough medical history is imperative with a cardiovascular patient, as it is with all handicapped patients. Inquiries pertaining to shortness of breath, high blood pressure, chest pains, swollen ankles, and the like may uncover an undiagnosed cardiac problem. Medical consultation with the patient's physician will assist you in treatment planning. Several medications prescribed for cardiovascular problems can influence the dental treatment. Anticoagulant therapy, for example, can interfere with proper clotting following an extraction. It is important to have the patient's physician adjust the dosage of anticoagulant prior to the surgical procedures. Other cardiovascular medications may interact unfavorably with conventional dental sedation techniques, requiring modification of these procedures.

Control of anxiety about dental treatment is especially important for the cardiovascular patient. An increased anxiety level can stress an already compromised cardiovascular system and trigger a medical emergency. The use of verbal relaxation techniques, such as those described in Chapter 6, can be helpful. These techniques, in combination with a preoperative sedative if necessary, help allay anxiety and allow dental treatment to proceed safely.

Patients with a history of congenital heart disease, rheumatic heart disease, or heart valve replacement require prophylactic antibiotics prior to dental therapy to prevent the development of a subacute bacterial endocarditis.

THE MEDICAL-DENTAL HISTORY

A medical history is a requirement for every patient who receives dental care through the private or institutionalized sector. The approaches to history taking, as well as the actual composition of a medical assessment, are limitless. Figure 11-1 presents a comprehensive health questionnaire detailing demographic data, review of systems, familial-social aspects, developmental information (for child patients), and dental history.

The extent and specificity of your history will be determined by your dentist employer, based on personal preference and type of service to be rendered. Nevertheless, you should have a voice in deciding the kind of history to be used, for at least two reasons. First, you will be the dental professional with whom the majority of patients will come in contact during their first office visit. Many patients are initially very reluctant to offer a complete exposition of their medical backgrounds. Your ability to communicate concern and empathy can encourage patients to disclose necessary medical information. At the same time, your patients will learn to trust you and respect the health education you have to offer them. Second, you must have a full understanding of the questions required by the history in order to be comfortable with

D
E
M
O
G
R
A
P
H
I
C

Name _____ Birthplace _____ Birthdate _____

Marital Status _____ Sex _____ Height _____ Weight _____

Address _____ Telephone _____

1. Are you under a physician's care? _____ Reason _____

   Physician's name _____ Address _____

   _____ Telephone _____

2. Are you taking any drugs, medicines or pills? _____

   What type? _____ Reason _____

3. Have you ever been hospitalized or required an operation? _____

   Reason _____

Do the following condition(s) apply to you?

S
Y
S
T
E
M
S

HEAD AND NECK	YES	NO
Visual impairments	__	__
Hearing impairments	__	__
Speech impairments	__	__
Headaches	__	__
Facial injuries	__	__
Pain in jaw, face, mouth	__	__
Tumors, growths, cysts or recurrent ulcers	__	__
Difficulty opening mouth, swallowing	__	__
Inability to smell, taste	__	__
Dry mouth, halitosis	__	__
Bleeding gums	__	__
Dizziness or vertigo	__	__
Explain _____		

CARDIOVASCULAR	YES	NO
Pain or pressure in chest	__	__
Heart rate irregularities	__	__
Heart murmur	__	__
Shortness of breath	__	__
High blood pressure	__	__
Swollen ankles or legs	__	__
Stroke	__	__
Frequent nose bleeds	__	__
Rheumatic fever	__	__
Explain _____		

RESPIRATORY	YES	NO
Difficulty breathing	__	__
Chronic hoarseness, cough	__	__
Continuous stuffynose, sinus	__	__
Tuberculosis	__	__
Asthma	__	__
Pneumonia	__	__
Explain _____		

GASTROINTESTINAL	YES	NO
Jaundice, hepatitis	__	__
Liver, gall bladder disease	__	__
Appetite problems	__	__
Frequent indigestion	__	__
Diarrhea or vomiting	__	__
Explain _____		

ENDOCRINE	YES	NO
Glandular, goiter or thyroid condition	__	__
Hot or cold sensitivity	__	__
Recent gain or loss of weight	__	__
Diabetes (patient or immediate family member)	__	__
Adrenal condition	__	__
Steroid therapy	__	__
Explain _____		

Figure 11.1 (page 1) A health history review guide useful in securing necessary medical and dental data for the patient with special needs.

your patients and to establish with them a rapport that will continue throughout care.

Dental professionals should utilize information obtained from physical, medical, and laboratory evaluations for the following important reasons:

To identify patients who have symptoms that may be representative of a serious, undetected disease that requires attention and/or might be complicated by dental treatment

SYSTEMS

FAMILY-SOCIAL

GENITOURINARY	YES	NO
Frequent urination	——	——
Cystitis	——	——
Kidney disease	——	——
Gout	——	——
Explain _____		

INTEGUMENT	YES	NO
Rash, hives	——	——
Acne	——	——
Skin discoloration	——	——
Tumors, growths or cysts	——	——
Explain _____		

NERVOUS	YES	NO
Gait irregularities	——	——
Epilepsy or convulsions	——	——
Shunt placement	——	——
Excessive nervousness	——	——
Ulcers, vomiting blood	——	——
Frequent fainting spells	——	——
Parasthesia, numbness or tingling sensations	——	——
Explain _____		

ALLERGIES	YES	NO
Hayfever	——	——
Series of injections	——	——
Antibiotics	——	——
Dental anesthetics	——	——
Foods	——	——
Other	——	——
Explain _____		

BLEEDING DISORDERS	YES	NO
Blood diseases	——	——
Hemophilia	——	——
Anemia	——	——
Blood transfusions	——	——
Bruise easily	——	——
Explain _____		

ORTHOPEDIC	YES	NO
Cortisone therapy	——	——
Fractures	——	——
Joint replacement	——	——
Pain or stiffness	——	——
Arthritis	——	——
Explain _____		

4. Do you have an alcohol, snuff or tobacco habit? _____

5. Do you have any inherited or congenital disorders? _____

6. Give brief statement of health status of immediate family, i.e. parents and siblings. _____

7. Do you or have you had any venereal diseases or other contagious conditions which we should be aware of? _____

8. (Women) Are you pregnant or have you been? _____ Number _____
    Complications _____ Menstrual or other gynecological problems _____

Figure 11.1 (page 2)

To identify patients who are taking medications or who have systemic disease or prostheses that may alter the course of dental treatment

To identify patients who are taking prescribed medication, which can alert you to the presence of an underlying disease that the patient may have failed to mention

To increase dental-medical communication, as well as patient–provider rapport

To protect the dental professional from legal risk[11]

D
E
N
T
A
L

9. Do you have a dentist? _____ When was your last visit? _____
    Did you receive an oral prophylaxis? _____ History of radiographs
    exposed? _____

10. Have you had any previous gum treatment? _____ Root canal therapy?
    _____ Extractions? _____ Orthodontic treatment? _____ Prosthetic
    appliances? _____

11. Do you feel your diet is well balanced? _____ Sucrose intake? _____
    Sodium intake? _____

12. Do you have any oral habits such as nail biting, grinding, etc.? ____
    _____

13. Do you possess any hereditary dental conditions? _____
    _____

14. Have your past dental experiences been pleasant? _____
    _____

15. Have you utilized any forms of fluoride currently or in the past? ___
    _____

16. Briefly describe your oral hygiene practices. _____
    _____

17. Do you presently have specific oral complaints of pain or discomfort?
    _____
    _____

Figure 11.1 (page 3)

THE MANAGEMENT OF MEDICAL EMERGENCIES

The best way to manage medical emergencies in the dental office is to prevent their occurrence! The first line of defense, as outlined in the preceding section, is to take a thorough medical history and to consult with all necessary medical personnel about medical abnormalities prior to initiating comprehensive oral rehabilitation.

Medical emergencies can occur despite the best preventive efforts, and you must, of course, be familiar with office policy and procedure. General initial management of a medical emergency is related to the *ABCs* of the American Heart Association—*airway, breathing,* and *circulation.*[12] Every member of the dental office staff should be certified in basic cardiopulmonary resuscitation techniques. Instruction in these techniques is available through local chapters of the American Heart Association.

Your ability to handle yourself appropriately in an emergency situation is as important as your knowledge of rescue techniques. You must appear calm and organized in your efforts to eliminate the patient's distress; otherwise, you will exacerbate the patient's anxiety and distress.

For a more thorough discussion of the management of specific medical emergencies, see *Clinical Practice of the Dental Hygienist.*[13]

CLINICAL EXAMINATIONS

Office Accessibility

The dental professional who decides to treat the patient with special needs must evaluate the physical architecture of the office to ensure that these patients will have easy access to the premises. Most offices can be made accessible with minimal effort and reasonable expense. Modifications include ramps and elevators, hallways and doors at least 30 to 36 inches wide, appropriate bathroom facilities, modern chairs, and portable equipment.[14]

Communication Skills

It is important to evaluate each patient's level of comprehension and the type of disability so that you can individualize your communication approach in order to maximize understanding of dental problems and their prevention.

Mental retardation.   The mentally retarded patient will require simple language and simple, specific instructions to ensure compliance. It is often necessary to repeat instructions several times. Multiple sessions to reinforce a particular task might be required, due to the limited attention span which often characterizes the retarded individual.

Mentally retarded patients often respond very well to praise. Praise should be used generously to reinforce appropriate behaviors as they occur during the course of the dental visit.

Cerebral palsy.   The patient with cerebral palsy is often of normal intelligence. Do not inadvertently insult the patient by assessing his level of comprehension on the basis of his physical disabilities and addressing him as if he were limited in intellectual ability.

If the patient is wheelchair-dependent, ask if he or she needs assistance in transferring to the dental chair; these patients often make the transfer better on their own. Communication should be aimed at relaxing the patient, because anxiety and tension increase involuntary movement. Your tone should be soothing and your pace relaxed.

The technique of Tell-Show-Do should be used to describe all dental procedures prior to initiating them to further reduce uncertainty and anxiety.[15] The Tell-Show-Do technique uses different methods of communication to describe each procedure. First, a verbal account of the procedure is provided (Tell); for example, explain to your patient the proper placement of the toothbrush bristles against the surfaces of the teeth. Next, demonstrate proper placement (Show) by using a large typodont and oversized toothbrush. Last, perform the procedure in the patient's mouth (Do).

Communication with the cerebral palsied patient can be complicated by the speech disturbances that are often associated with this disorder. In such cases, assistance from a parent or companion can be valuable. Finally, we recommend the use of shorter appointments for the patient with cerebral palsy in order to help reduce agitated muscle spasms brought on by fatigue.[16]

Seizure disorders.   Stress can trigger convulsive episodes in the seizure-disordered patient. The Tell-Show-Do method can be used to reduce anxiety, as can verbal relaxation techniques. It is important not to startle the patient by the unannounced use of dental equipment or instruments (such as the dental handpiece, dental light, or amalgamator).

If the patient has a seizure while in the dental chair, do not panic. Protect the patient from falling and from potentially harmful instruments or equipment. Turn the patient on his side to prevent aspiration of secretions, loosen clothing about the neck, and be prepared to administer oxygen. Do not attempt to force the teeth apart, even if the tongue has been bitten, because of the potential for further injury to the oral cavity as a result of such action. The patient may require assistance and reassurance after the seizure episode.

Oncology.   Patients with cancer of the head and neck region who are undergoing radiation therapy or chemotherapy must be given extensive dental health education. It is extremely important to convey the importance of oral maintenance not only to the patient, but also to the medical professionals responsible for the patient's treatment (including the oncologist, radiologist, and surgeon). Too often, the dental practitioner is consulted after the onset of therapy, when stomatotoxicity is already apparent or questionable teeth require extraction. Communication between members of the medical and dental professions must begin during the period following diagnosis of the patient's condition, prior to the onset of therapy. This will enable the dental practitioner to provide the cancer patient with an asymptomatic, functioning oral environment ultimately free of infection or other complications that may induce an exaggerated response when medical treatment is introduced.[9]

Informing the patient honestly of the oral complications associated with therapy and the preventive measures that can be taken to reduce their chances of occurrence is of the utmost importance. Encourage the patient to visit frequently so that you can assess his oral status and make yourself available to meet his needs.

Sensory impairments.   Although blindness is a severe handicap, the visually disabled patient should pose few problems for the dental professional if there are no additional handicapping conditions. Explain all procedures and equipment carefully. Postural changes such as adjustment of the dental chair should be announced in advance. The Tell-Show-Do method is appropriate, but the Show aspect must be accomplished using nonvisual (tactile or auditory) cues. The patient's age at onset of blindness will determine the extent to which you can make verbal comparisons with shapes, colors, and textures. If a patient lost his sight during the teenage years, for example, he will be able to comprehend the color red when you describe disclosing solution or inflamed gingiva.

The deaf patient can present quite a communication challenge, because the standard verbal approach is severely limited. The type and severity of the disability and the method of communication used by the patient must be considered when attempting to establish an adequate dialogue.

If the patient reads lips, be sure that you maintain face-to-face contact. Do not exaggerate sounds, however, as this will tend to confuse, rather than enhance, comprehension. Some deaf patients have been taught manual communication. If you are not familiar with sign language, it will be necessary to have an interpreter present during treatment. Useful signs for the dental professional are illustrated in an article by Mueller and Gantt.[17]

If all else fails, writing with a pad and pencil can be used as a major means of communication. Drawings on cards (made in advance of the appointment) can be helpful for explaining procedures.[18] Deaf patients can also benefit from observing other patients being treated in the office; such observation serves to enhance understanding and acceptance of dental treatment.

The multiply handicapped patient who is both deaf and blind poses additional obstacles to dental management. If you are unable to establish an avenue of communication with such a patient, dental habilitation may require pharmacotherapeutic control with premedication or general anesthesia.

Cardiovascular.   Cardiovascular disease is one of the most frequently encountered handicapping conditions in the dental office. It is imperative that you consult with the patient's physician before beginning dental treatment. The reduction of anxiety is, as we have noted, essential in order to minimize potential complications. The dental professional's knowledge of the specific condition, the medications taken, and the need for prophylactic antibiotic coverage is necessary for optimal management of the patient with cardiovascular disease.

Scheduling

Scheduling is important if the patient with special needs is to be efficiently treated. If the patient is taking medication, it is often necessary to arrange the dental appointment to coincide with the period during which the medication is of optimal efficacy. For example, it would be advantageous to schedule a seizure-disordered patient 1 to 2 hours following ingestion of the first morning dose of medication. The diabetic patient is best appointed in the morning following breakfast. Be sure to ask these patients if they have taken their medication.

The physically disabled patient might require more time than is usually necessary to prepare for a dental appointment. These patients often need additional time for personal hygiene, eating, and traveling. It would be inappropriate and uncaring to schedule these patients for the first or second appointment of the day. A late morning or early afternoon appointment would probably be more suitable. Of course, you should attempt to schedule handicapped patients at a time during the day that is conducive to efficient dental care delivery. Certain patients undergo mood fluctuations during the course of the day, so the appointment for such a patient should coincide with a positive period, if possible.

The length of appointments is another factor to consider when scheduling. The mentally retarded individual with a limited attention span would be better treated in multiple, short appointments than in one or two long, tiresome appointments. Cerebral palsied patients also benefit from shorter appointments because of the problems associated with motor control. Intervals between appointments must also be considered. The cardiac patient who requires antibiotic coverage to prevent subacute bacterial endocarditis, for example, should be scheduled to allow at least 2 weeks between appointments, in order to reduce the prevalence of resistant bacterial strains.

Assessment Devices and Radiographic Techniques

It is often necessary to utilize mouth-opening devices in order to efficiently treat handicapped patients. Figure 11-2 depicts several devices that have proven useful in dental treatment. If it becomes necessary to use such a device, inform the patient that the device is necessary in order to keep the mouth in an open position with minimum fatigue.

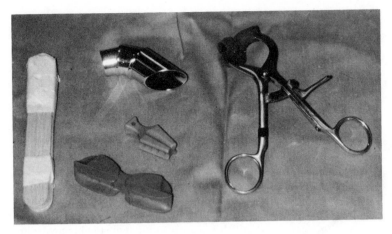

Figure 11.2 Several mouth-opening devices for maintaining access to the oral cavity during examination, preventive procedures, or oral rehabilitation.

The patient should never feel that the use of the device is a punitive measure to obtain compliance.

In order to gather all necessary diagnostic data, you will often have to modify standard procedures to accommodate the patient with special needs. Radiographic evaluation of the dentition and supporting structures is an integral part of the clinical examination, and every effort should be made to secure diagnostic films.

Although taking dental radiographs is a fairly innocuous procedure, many handicapped patients will not permit you to proceed in a conventional manner. While many of these patients will discourage placement of an intraoral film, they will readily accept an extraoral approach. Panoramic radiography (Figure 11-3) and a 450-degree oblique

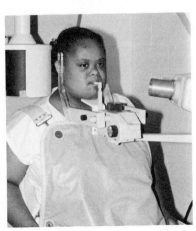

Figure 11.3 Demonstration of panoramic radiographic technique.

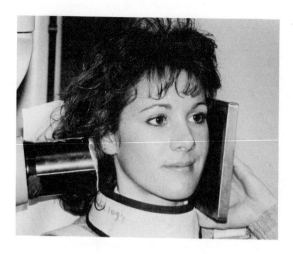

Figure 11.4 Placement of the film cassette during extraoral radiographic procedures.

film cassette (Figure 11-4) are two modified radiographic procedures which require minimal cooperation on the part of the patient.

If the patient presents with an exaggerated gag reflex but readily accepts intraoral placement of a dental film, placing the film in the buccal vestibule instead of against the tongue can allow a modified bite-wing radiograph to be exposed (Figure 11-5).

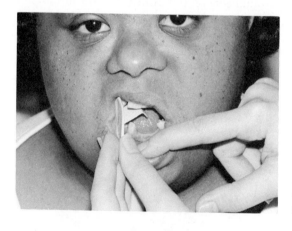

Figure 11.5   Demonstration of intraoral reverse bitewing technique.

PREVENTIVE ORAL HYGIENE

Positioning

For the patient with special needs, oral hygiene procedures frequently must be accomplished by the individual responsible for the patient's general care. Two factors must be considered in order to effectively proceed with oral hygiene care: visibility and behavior control.

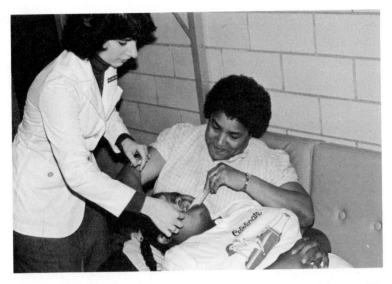

Figure 11.6 The dental hygienist describing and demonstrating modifications in oral hygiene techniques.

Figure 11-6 shows the dental hygienist explaining proper positioning to a parent and daughter. Notice the visibility of and ease of access to the oral cavity enabled by having the patient rest her head on her mother's lap. The use of a couch, bed, or even the floor can be advantageous.

The position demonstrated in Figure 11-7 might be necessary for

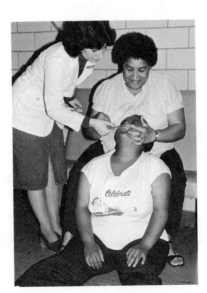

Figure 11.7 The dental hygienist explaining to the caretaker a position that will increase visibility and access to the oral cavity and control extraneous movements.

the patient with many arm or leg movements. Control is obtained by the placement of the caretaker's legs over the patient's shoulders.

Patients with cerebral palsy often exhibit grotesque muscular contortions. Dental treatment for such a patient is often more easily accomplished by placing him in a bean bag chair on top of the dental chair. The bodily support and containment provided minimizes movement, but success with this approach has been limited to child patients.[18]

Individualized Oral Hygiene Techniques

Mental retardation.   The mentally retarded patient might experience motor difficulties such as a hyperactive gag reflex or poor tongue control. This, in combination with impaired cognitive functioning, can prove quite challenging to the dental professional who is attempting to teach general oral hygiene procedures.

Oral hygiene programs for the retarded patient should involve the patient and the caretaker. The retarded patient's oral hygiene care is often neglected as a result of preoccupation with the physical and mental disabilities. Excessive use of the bottle and of cariogenic reinforcers for appropriate behavior—especially in institutions—contributes greatly to the incidence of dental caries.

When you plan an oral hygiene program for the retarded patient, progress slowly. Rehearse each technique with the patient until he has mastered it, with or without the aid of the caretaker. Do not hold unrealistic expectations for these patients; recognize their limitations. Praise the patient continuously, and reinforce desirable behavior with small material rewards such as stars and stickers. Be creative in your approach to care.

The toothbrush modifications illustrated in Figure 11-8 can be

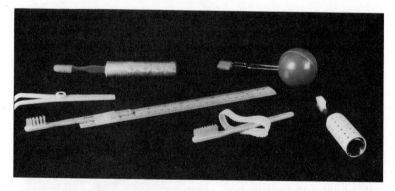

Figure 11.8 A variety of modified oral hygiene aids designed for the patient with neuromuscular impairment.

helpful with the retarded patient who is able to brush but who has some motor problems.

Cerebral palsy.   The toothbrush modifications shown in Figure 11-8 are ideally suited for use with the patient with cerebral palsy. The extended and enlarged handles serve to accommodate patients with impaired motor coordination, and they can be constructed easily and inexpensively. Mouth-propping devices are often required to retain the mouth in an open position during oral hygiene care (Figure 11-9). The fabrication of a suction toothbrush is also advised for use with patients who have excessive salivary secretions.[13] Use your ingenuity to develop aids to meet your patients' individual needs.

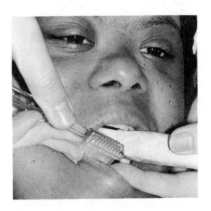

Figure 11.9 Demonstration of a tongue blade mouth prop incorporated into an oral hygiene home care program.

The cerebral palsied patient often exhibits inadequate control of the oral musculature, which encourages collection of food debris and bacterial plaque. Excessive drooling due to hypotonicity of the lip muscles and the predominance of mouth breathing fosters increased production of calculus and gingival inflammation.[18] Dietary considerations are also necessary; because motor impairments discourage consumption of fibrous foods, the patient is likely to be consuming more highly processed foods which are high in sucrose.

Recommendations must be made concerning toothbrushing, daily fluoride gel applications, semisoft diet alternatives, oral physical therapy, and frequent dental visits to monitor progress.

Seizure disorders.   Oral hygiene is the major component of dental care for the seizure-disordered patient who is managed with Dilantin. The gingival hyperplasia seen in these patients is the result of an exaggerated response to the presence of plaque and other gingival irritants in combination with drug therapy. The gingival overgrowth appears pale and fibrotic.

Meticulous oral hygiene is necessary to maintain the size, texture, and contour of the gingiva. If pseudopockets are the result of this overgrowth and the gingival tissue partially or completely covers the teeth, gingival surgery may be required. This is not a cure, however, and hyperplasia will recur if oral hygiene measures are less than optimal.

Oncology.   Oral hygiene is a top priority for the patient who is undergoing radiation therapy for a tumor of the head or neck region and for the cancer patient who requires chemotherapy. The radiation patient may exhibit side effects such as xerostomia, mucositis, trismus, difficulty swallowing, altered taste, and sensitivity to pressure or temperature. If the salivary glands are in the site of the x-ray beam, the glands may atrophy, altering the salivary flow and producing xerostomia. The viscous, highly acidic saliva increases the patient's susceptibility to dental caries. Mucositis involves a sloughing of the oral mucosa. Because the outer stratified squamous nonkeratinized epithelium is being destroyed, the underlying, fragile oral mucosa is exposed, leaving the mouth extremely sensitive and susceptible to disruption by mechanical or bacterial invasion.

The oral care regimen should include the following:

1. An immaculate oral cavity to prevent periodontal infection
2. Daily fluoride applications
3. A low-sucrose diet
4. Oral physical therapy to prevent or treat trismus
5. Artificial salivas for xerostomia
6. Avoidance of smoking, alcohol, or commercial mouthwashes, due to their irritating effect on the oral mucosa

Of these steps, numbers 2 and 3 will reduce the patient's susceptibility to dental caries; numbers 1, 2, and 3 will reduce the patient's risk of developing osteoradionecrosis.

Oral side effects are potentially lethal for the patient who is undergoing chemotherapy. These side effects include mucositis, ulcerations, infection, xerostomia, and spontaneous bleeding. Chemotherapy involves the use of drugs that function by suppressing the growth and spread of malignant cells. Unfortunately, normal cells are also adversely affected during the course of treatment. Normal cells that have the highest rate of mitotic activity—cells of the mouth, digestive tract, bone marrow, hair follicles, and reproductive system—are directly affected by chemotherapy through an interference in cell production, maturation, and replacement. Consequently, oral mucositis, ulcerations, and xerostomia may develop. Indirect toxicity is caused by the myelo-suppressive action of the drugs, resulting in a generalized immuno-suppression; neutropenia, lymphocytopenia, and thrombocytopenia will make the patient very susceptible to infection and spontaneous bleeding.

Systematic oral hygiene care has been shown to decrease the incidence of oral complications. Prepare a protocol for these patients to meet their specific needs. Close attention should be paid to frequent oral examinations, palliative measures directed toward side effects as they arise, meticulous oral hygiene, diet, and fluctuations in the patient's blood cell levels, particularly platelet and white blood cell counts.[9]

Vision impaired.   When one loses the sense of sight, the senses of touch, taste, smell, and hearing become very acute. These senses should be utilized to their fullest capacity during the dental health education experience. Since the patient is unable to learn by visual imitation, explicit verbal instructions become extremely important. Verbal instructions should incorporate textures, contours, odors, vibrations and pulsations, light or heavy pressures, and wetness or dryness.[19]

The patient should demonstrate his brushing technique at the outset of the appointment. Although the patient cannot benefit from observing the effects of disclosing solution, it can help you to assess the patient's plaque control techniques. Be careful and accurate in describing missed areas to the patient. Place the patient's finger on each problem area, describing it in relation to other teeth. The actual cleansing of these problem areas can be accomplished by guiding the patient's hand as he brushes. Establishing a brushing routine will help ensure plaque control effectiveness. Musical programs to teach sequential toothbrushing are available.[20]

Hearing impaired.   The ideal method for providing dental health education to the hearing impaired patient is through demonstration. Effective use of mirrors, models, drawings, and written forms of communication are invaluable tools. Disclosing solution is probably the best agent for promoting effective oral hygiene habits.

Cardiovascular.   As previously mentioned, many of your patients with cardiovascular disease are likely to require prophylactic antibiotics prior to oral prophylaxis. Routine oral hygiene is of particular importance to the patient who suffers from congenital or rheumatic heart disease, who requires heart surgery, or who has prosthetic heart valves.[21]

Bacteremias can result from exploration during an oral exam. Organisms can enter the bloodstream through a diseased sulcus or pocket while the patient is eating or during an oral prophylaxis. The greater the degree of periodontal involvement, the greater the patient's susceptibility to bacteremia. Hence, obtain a thorough medical history to determine the need for antibiotic coverage before evaluating your patient's oral health. The high-risk patient should be given initial oral hygiene instructions while he is under antibiotic coverage; then the teeth can be managed periodontally. Research shows that the risk of inducing a bacteremia through oral hygiene practices are reduced if the oral tissues are healthy. Avoid any unnecessary trauma that could provide a portal of entry for bacteria.

INSTITUTIONAL CARE

The practice of preventive dentistry and the role of the dental hygienist in a state facility is often different from what one might be accustomed to in a private setting. Because state facilities have limited financial resources, the dental hygienist is sometimes charged with the responsibility for administrating the hospital's total dental program. The hygienist might be responsible for ordering all necessary dental armamentarium, overseeing a preventive dental health education program, and monitoring the dental status of each resident at the institution. The multiplicity of roles and responsibilities in such a situation demands good communication skills, because the dental hygienist must be able to educate physicians, nursing staff, hospital administrators, and other health professionals concerning the importance of good oral health.[22]

The implementation of a total dental health program at a state facility can be separated into three components, the first of which is the establishment of a dental training program for auxiliary personnel. After extensive instruction, they should be able to perform daily oral hygiene tasks for each resident. The second component involves the education of the dietary staff and the psychologists employed at the institution. During this phase, the dental hygienist should describe the etiology of dental disease, highlighting the importance of sucrose in the disease process. Attempts should be made to decrease sucrose consumption both in amount and frequency. The psychologists should be encouraged to substitute noncariogenic foods as rewards for appropriate behavior. The final component of a total dental program involves securing comprehensive oral rehabilitation for each resident who requires such services. In order to ensure that each resident's dental needs are properly met, it might be necessary to canvas local dental practitioners if there are no dentists on the hospital staff.

REFERENCES

1. Public Health Service. Health characteristics of persons with chronic activity limitations—U.S., 1974. U.S. Vital and Health Statistics Series 10. U.S. Department of Health, Education, and Welfare. Government Printing Office, Washington, D.C., 1976.

2. Nowak, A.J. *Dentistry for the handicapped patient.* St. Louis: C.V. Mosby, 1976.

3. Miller, S.L. Dental care for the mentally retarded: A challenge to the profession. *Journal of Public Health Dentistry* 25:3, 1965.

4. Stiefel, D.J. Inclusion of a program of instruction in care of the disabled in a dental school curriculum. *Journal of Dental Education* 43:262, 1979.

5. The Robert Wood Johnson Foundation. News Release, June 22, 1973.

6. Pinkham, J.R. The handicapped patient. In *Textbook of pediatric dentistry.* Edited by R.L. Braham and M.E. Morris. Baltimore: Williams and Wilkins, 1980.

7. Kamen, S. Mental retardation. In *Dentistry for the handicapped.* Edited by A.J. Nowak. St. Louis: C.V. Mosby, 1976.

8. Sorenson, H.W. Physically handicapped. In *Dentistry for the handicapped.* Edited by A.J. Nowak. St. Louis: C.V. Mosby, 1976.

9. DeBiase, C.B., and Komives, B.K. An oral care protocol for leukemic patients with chemotherapy-induced complications. *Special Care in Dentistry* 3:207, 1983.

10. Kanar, H.L. The blind and the deaf. In *Dentistry for the handicapped.* Edited by A.J. Nowak. St. Louis: C.V. Mosby, 1976.

11. Little, J.W., and Falace, D.A. *Dental management of the medically compromised patient.* St. Louis: C.V. Mosby, 1980.

12. American Heart Association. Standards and guidelines for cardiopulmonary rescuscitation and emergency. *Journal of the American Medical Association* 244:453, 1980.

13. Wilkins, E.M. *Clinical practice of the dental hygienist,* 5th ed. Philadelphia: Lea and Febiger, 1983.

14. Gutman, E.M. *Wheelchair to independence: Architectural barriers eliminated.* Springfield, Ill.: Charles C. Thomas, 1968.

15. Addelston, H.K. Child patient training. *Fortnightly Review of the Chicago Dental Society* 38:7, 1959.

16. Spencer, P.R. The role of the dental assistant in the management of the handicapped patient. *Dental Clinics of North America* 18:633, 1974.

17. Mueller, K., and Gantt, D. Communicating with the deaf patient. *Journal of Dentistry for the Handicapped* 3:22, 1978.

18. Lange, B.M., Entwistle, B.M., and Lipson, L.F. *Dental management for the handicapped: Approaches for dental auxiliaries.* Philadelphia: Lea and Febiger, 1983.

19. Engar, R.C., and Stiefel, D.J. *Dental treatment for the sensory impaired patient.* Disability Dental Instruction. Seattle, Wash.: University of Washington School of Dentistry, 1977.

20. Clemens, C., and Taylor, S. Toothbrushing to music. *Dental Hygiene* 54:125, 1980.

21. American Heart Association. Prevention of bacterial endocarditis. *Journal of the American Dental Association* 95:600, 1977.

22. Fenton, S.J., DeBiase, C.B., and Portugal, B.V. A strategy for implementing a dental health education program for state facilities with limited resources. *Rehabilitation Literature* 43:290, 1982.

Appendix A:
Relaxation Instructions

The method of relaxation training we think you will find most helpful is actually a composite of several approaches. The use of tension-relaxation cycles with major muscle groups is drawn from the work of Joseph Wolpe,[1] who based his technique on the methods developed by Edmund Jacobson.[2] This method, known as *progressive relaxation*, has been shown to lower resting levels of muscle tension and autonomic arousal.

Relaxation, as both a process and a state, involves more than simply reducing muscular tension, however: There is also a cognitive/emotional component that includes feelings of well-being and a sense of peace and comfort. To promote and enhance these feelings, we have included suggestions and imagery that have been developed by our colleagues in the field of clinical hypnosis.* These experienced therapists, many of whom were trained by Milton Erickson, do not attempt to direct or bend a patient's behavior to fit their own expectations of how the patient should behave or what he should experience. Instead, they believe that the patient's own unconscious has the skills and ability to solve the problem, so they see their task as simply helping the patient to focus his attention in order to discover and utilize the skills he already possesses.

*We gratefully acknowledge Doctors Kay Thompson, Robert Pearson, and Bertha Roger.

From a clinical point of view, this approach makes very good sense. If the therapist does all the work for the patient by telling him exactly what to feel, imagine, and experience, then it is the therapist, not the patient, who is in control. At best, even if the patient succeeds in following these instructions, he will credit the therapist with the successful outcome (in this case, a state of deep relaxation) and will have little faith in his ability to reproduce the results on his own. At worst—because many people do not like to be told what to do—the patient will sabotage the therapist's efforts, without consciously intending to do so, and will not have a successful experience.

Therefore, in addition to the more rigidly structured muscle relaxation exercises, we have included a less structured approach to helping the patient achieve a state of deep relaxation and comfort through the use of imagery. We think that this combination of more and less structured approaches is particularly well suited for use in a standardized audiotaped format. Further, it is a method that can be effectively employed by the dental professional who has no formal training in psychology.

INSTRUCTIONS

To make a relaxation tape for use by patients, follow the script (below). Note that the italicized material is intended as instructions to you and should not be included on the tape.

Speak in a calm, soothing tone and keep your pace steady and unhurried. Allow a few moments of silence at the beginning of the tape and several minutes more at the end.

SCRIPT

Learning how to relax does not really involve learning anything new, because your body already knows how to relax and feel comfortable. Most people, for example, can recall the pleasant sensations of lying on a beach in the warm sun. Or maybe you can remember how comfortable it feels to curl up in front of a cozy fire on a cold winter night. You can learn to recall these good feelings of relaxation and comfort and actually experience them any time you choose.

To help you recall the feeling of muscular relaxation, we will begin by asking you to alternately tense and relax various groups of muscles in your body. As you tense each group of muscles, you can be aware of the feelings and sensations that accompany muscular tension. Then, as you turn off the tension and let the muscles relax, it is interesting to notice the difference. There is no need to force the relaxation: You can just be curious as you allow the muscles to recall the sensation of being loose, limp, and completely relaxed.

We will begin with your hands and arms; then we will focus on the muscles in your face and scalp; next, your back, shoulders, and abdomen; and finally, we will focus on your legs and feet.

The words "Now tense" will be your cue to tense the muscles. By allowing the rest of your body to remain relaxed and comfortable, you will be able to focus your attention directly on the area of tension.

The words "Now relax" will be your signal to turn off the tension and let go. Some people like to think of turning off a switch and letting the tension go as suddenly and completely as the lights go out when you turn off a light switch. It can be interesting, just letting go: Even when you think the tension is gone, let go even further—perhaps you can actually feel the tension draining out and away from the muscles as the comfortable feelings of relaxation proceed on their own. Let's begin with your right hand.

1. *Right Hand*
   a. *Tension* At the signal "Now tense," make a fist with your right hand. Remember to allow the rest of your body to remain relaxed as you focus your attention on the tension in your right hand, fingers, and wrist. Now tense. *(10-second pause)*
   b. *Relaxation (Allow pause of approximately 10 seconds at each *)* Good. Now relax. Let go of all the tension in your right hand. Allow the fingers to become limp and loose. (*) Notice how comfortable these muscles feel as the tension drains out and away. (*) Continue to let the tension flow down and out through the tips of your fingers. (*)

2. *Right Arm*
   a. *Tension* At the signal "Now tense," tense the biceps in your right arm by pushing your right elbow down against the chair. Now tense. *(10-second pause)*
   b. *Relaxation (Allow pause of approximately 10 seconds at each *)* Fine. Now relax. Turn off the tension in these muscles. Just let go. (*) Your arm can become as loose and as limp as an old piece of rope just tossed on the ground (*) Can that arm become even more relaxed? (*)

3. *Left Hand*
   (Repeat a and b of Right Hand, substituting words "left hand")

4. *Left Arm*
   (Repeat a and b of Right Arm, substituting words "left arm")

5. *Forehead and Scalp*

   a. *Tension* At the signal "Now tense," make the muscles in your forehead and scalp tense by raising your eyebrows as high as you can. Now tense. *(10-second pause)*

   b. *Relaxation (Allow pause of approximately 10 seconds at each *)* Good. Now relax. Let your eyebrows return comfortably to their natural position. Let your forehead and scalp smooth out and let the relaxation spread. (*) Notice how comfortable these muscles feel as the tension drains away. (*) Let the muscles become looser and looser. (*)

6. *Eyes, Nose (Omit if tape is to be used by patients during dental procedures)*

   a. *Tension* At the signal "Now tense," produce tension around your eyes and nose by squinting your eyes tightly shut and wrinkling up your nose. Now tense. *(10-second pause)*

   b. *Relaxation (Allow pause of approximately 10 seconds at each *)* Fine. Now relax. Turn off the tension, just like turning off a light switch. (*) Let the muscles in your face fall into a natural, comfortable position. (*) The relaxation can proceed on its own. (*)

7. *Mouth, Jaws (Omit if tape is to be used by patients during dental procedures)*

   a. *Tension* At the signal "Now tense," clench your teeth tightly together and press your tongue against the roof of your mouth. Remember to allow the rest of your body to remain relaxed and at ease. Now tense. *(10-second pause)*

   b. *Relaxation (Allow pause of approximately 10 seconds at each *)* Very good. And now relax. Your jaws and your tongue can assume a more comfortable position and the tension can melt away. (*) No effort is necessary—it can happen naturally, with no work on your part. Your jaws and your tongue can remember how to feel comfortable. (*) As the tension melts away, the relaxation can proceed on its own. (*)

8. *Neck*

   a. *Tension* At the signal "Now tense," push your head gently back against the chair so that you feel tension in your neck. The rest of your body can remain relaxed and comfortable. Now tense. *(10-second pause)*

   b. *Relaxation (Allow pause of approximately 10 seconds at each *)* Excellent. And now relax. As you turn off these muscles, you can allow your head to feel pleasantly heavy. Let it rest comfortably against the chair. (*) You can be interested in the sensations in these muscles. (*) You wonder just how heavy and comfortable your head and your neck can feel. (*)

9. *Shoulders, Upper Back*

   a. *Tension* At the signal "Now tense," pull your shoulder blades together in the back. Let the rest of your body remain relaxed so that you can focus your attention on the tension in your shoulders and your upper back. Now tense. *(10-second pause)*

   b. *Relaxation (Allow pause of approximately 10 seconds at each *)* That's fine. Now relax. Let your shoulders drop into a natural, relaxed position and let the tension drain out of your shoulders and your back. (*) Perhaps you notice that your arms feel more comfortable when your shoulders and back are relaxed. (*) Just let your body remember how pleasant and comfortable it can feel.

10. *Abdomen*

    a. *Tension* At the signal "Now tense," make your stomach muscles very tense. Now tense. Notice that it is difficult to breathe easily when these muscles are tense and strained. *(10-second pause)*

    b. *Relaxation (Allow pause of approximately 10 seconds at each *)* Fine. Now relax. Let the muscles in your stomach become loose and relaxed. (*) Enjoy the sensation of breathing easily and freely, in and out. (*) Each time you exhale, you can let these muscles relax a little more. (*)

11. *Right Thigh*

    a. *Tension* At the signal "Now tense," tense the large muscle on top of your right thigh. Pay attention to the feelings of tension. Now tense. *(10-second pause)*

    b. *Relaxation (Allow pause of approximately 10 seconds at each *)* Very good. Now relax. Just as you can turn off a light switch, you can turn off tension in any muscle in your body. (*) As you continue to let go, your leg can feel heavy and limp. (*) It can be an enjoyable sensation. (*)

12. *Right Calf*

    a. *Tension* At the signal "Now tense," create tension in the muscles of your right calf by pulling your toes up toward your head. Now tense. *(10-second pause)*

    b. *Relaxation (Allow pause of approximately 10 seconds at each *)* That's good. Now relax. Let your foot fall into a relaxed, easy position and let the muscles become loose and limp. (*) Your muscles can recall the sensation of being quiet, comfortable, and at rest. (*) The relaxation can continue to grow deeper and deeper. (*)

13. *Right Foot*
   a. *Tension* At the signal "Now tense," curl the toes on your right foot under to create feelings of tension in your foot. Focus on the tension. Now tense. *(10-second pause)*
   b. *Relaxation (Allow pause of approximately 10 seconds at each *)* Very nice. Now relax. As you uncurl your toes, you can turn off the muscles and let your foot become as relaxed as it needs to be to feel very comfortable. (*) Very easy, very nice. (*) You might notice a feeling of heaviness in your foot and your leg as the relaxation spreads and deepens. (*)

14. *Left Thigh*
   (Repeat a and b of Right Thigh, substituting words "left thigh")

15. *Left Calf*
   (Repeat a and b of Right Calf, substituting words "left calf")

16. *Left Foot*
   (Repeat a and b of Right Foot, substituting words "left foot")

As your body becomes more comfortable, you might notice different sensations. Perhaps you will feel very heavy as you sink down into a state of quiet comfort. *(10-second pause)* Or maybe you will experience a pleasant feeling of lightness, as if you were floating. *(10-second pause)* As your hands and your arms and your neck and your shoulders become more and more comfortable, you can be curious about what pleasant feelings you can experience. *(10-second pause)*

Perhaps you have noticed that your breathing has become calm and quiet as your body becomes still and peaceful. *(10-second pause)* And it is possible to become even more comfortable simply by taking a deep breath, then exhaling very slowly as you allow yourself to let go. *(30-second pause)*

As you enjoy these pleasant sensations, I wonder if you can allow yourself to recall similar feelings of comfort. Perhaps you have experienced such feelings on a beach, lying in the warm sun. *(30-second pause)* Some people might recall a quiet autumn afternoon in the woods and fields. *(30-second pause)* Or a happy time many years ago. *(30-second pause)* Or even something in the future. *(30-second pause)* You will know the things you like best.

REFERENCES

1. Wolpe, J. *Psychotherapy by reciprocal inhibition.* Stanford, California: Stanford University Press, 1958.
2. Jacobson, E. *Progressive relaxation.* Chicago: University of Chicago Press, 1938.

Appendix B:
Dental Fear Hierarchy

As discussed in Chapter 6, the process of systematic desensitization involves presenting the relaxed patient with a series of imaginal scenes, rank-ordered from least to most threatening or fear arousing. In clinical practice, the therapist and patient work together to develop a list of scenes, and the patient rank-orders them according to how frightening each is to him. Of course, this cannot be done when you are making a taped desensitization program. For most fearful dental patients, however, the feared situation and the relative amount of threat each represents are sufficiently similar across patients that a standard hierarchy can be employed.

A standard dental fear hierarchy is presented below. Each item should be presented for 30 to 60 seconds. The patient is then instructed to stop visualizing the scene and to simply relax for 30 to 60 seconds. The scene is then repeated for 30 to 60 seconds, followed again by 30 to 60 seconds of relaxation.

FEAR HIERARCHY

1. You are calling to make a dental appointment. First you look up the telephone number. Then you dial the telephone. It rings three or four times and the receptionist answers. You tell her your name, describe your problem, and tell her that you would like to make an appointment. You agree on an appointment for the following week.

2. It is the morning of your dental appointment. You think about the fact that you will be in the dental chair in a few hours, and the thought makes you feel a little uneasy. You say to yourself, "Well, it's probably not going to be so bad," and you feel better.

3. You leave for your appointment. You drive to the dentist's office and look for a place to park. You feel a little uncomfortable but you are sure that you can handle it.

4. You leave your car and walk toward the office. You take the elevator to the correct floor and walk down the hall to the office.

5. You open the door and walk into the office. The receptionist looks up to greet you. You give your name and take a seat.

6. You are seated in the waiting room, reading a magazine. There are two or three other people in the room. The dental assistant appears in the doorway and calls your name.

7. You greet the assistant and proceed into the dental operatory. As you walk toward the chair, you begin to feel a little nervous. You seat yourself in the chair, take a deep breath, exhale slowly, and sink back. You notice that the chair is really rather comfortable.

8. When the dentist enters, you smile and say hello. He asks how you have been and you chat for a minute or two. He washes his hands and seats himself beside the dental chair. He asks how he can help you and you tell him about the problem you've been having. He listens carefully and nods. He asks you some questions and says, "I see."

9. The dentist asks you to open your mouth. He picks up a small mirror and a probe and asks you to point to the problem area. The dentist probes gently. You feel a little tense as you feel the probe against your gums, but you know that the most you will experience is a little discomfort. You close your eyes and allow your body to remember to be comfortable and relaxed.

10. The dentist tells you that you have some decay where part of an old filling has fallen out. He tells you that he would like to remove the old filling and the decay, then replace the filling. You don't much like the idea of drilling, but you say you are glad he can save the tooth. The dentist smiles and says, "So am I."

11. The dentist prepares the anesthetic injection. You feel uneasy because the thought of an injection makes you a little nervous. You know, however, that you will only feel a pinch, and that the idea of the injection is worse than the injection itself.

12. The dentist asks you to open your mouth. You decide it will be easier if you relax. You close your eyes, take a deep breath, and allow your body to become loose and limp. It feels rather nice to

be so relaxed. You feel a pinch and a sting. Then the dentist says, "Okay, that's fine." You feel pleased because it really didn't bother you very much.

13. Your mouth feels numb in the area around the problem tooth, and the dentist is ready to begin. Before he begins, you tell him that you will signal him by raising your hand if you want him to stop at any time. He says "Fine." This makes you feel a bit more comfortable, because you know that you are in control.

14. The dentist is drilling your tooth. You hear the sound of the high-speed drill and you feel the vibration in your mouth. You are feeling rather bored and begin to think about your plans for an upcoming holiday weekend.

15. The dentist pauses to examine your tooth. He nods and says, "Um-hm, that looks good." The dental assistant begins to mix the material for the filling.

16. The dentist puts the filling material in place and packs it firmly. He works on your tooth with several instruments. You are relieved that he is almost finished because you are beginning to feel a bit sleepy.

17. The dentist asks you to bite down gently. He checks the tooth and makes an adjustment. Then he says, "There, all finished." You get up, say goodbye, and leave. You feel a little tired, but calm and relaxed. You arrange for your next appointment, say goodbye to the receptionist, and leave the office.

Index